MANAGE
YOUR PAIN

ABOUT THE AUTHORS

Assoc. Prof. Michael Nicholas, PhD

Michael has been working in the pain field since 1980 as a clinical psychologist, educator, and researcher. Between 1988 and 1990 Michael was the inaugural director of the inpatient pain management programme (INPUT) at St Thomas' Hospital in London. This programme was established with the support of the Kings Fund to evaluate the effectiveness of this form of pain management in the UK. The INPUT programme continues to achieve outstanding results and over the years it has received widespread international recognition. Since returning to Australia Michael joined the Pain Management and Research Centre at the Royal North Shore Hospital in Sydney (with the Faculty of Medicine, University of Sydney), where he is now an Associate Professor. In 1994 Michael established the ADAPT programme at the Royal North Shore Hospital. This is based directly on the original INPUT programme in London and is achieving similar results. More recently, he has been involved in assisting the development of similar programmes in Malaysia, Hong Kong, the Philippines and Singapore, as well as Australia. Michael has published over 120 papers in books and scientific journals, on the management of pain, and he has lectured on the field in many countries.

Dr Allan Molloy

Allan is a graduate of The Middlesex Hospital Medical School, University of London, where he was also awarded a BSc (Hons) in Neuropharmacology. After training at Addenbrookes Hospital, Cambridge, the Bristol Royal Infirmary, St. Bartholomew's Hospital and Great Ormond Street Hospital, London, he qualified as an Anaesthetist in 1992. He then moved to Australia to further his training in pain management, and is now a Senior Lecturer and Senior Specialist at the Pain Management and Research Centre at the Royal North Shore Hospital in Sydney (with the Faculty of Medicine, University of Sydney). Allan is a Foundation Fellow of the Faculty of Pain Medicine, Australian and New Zealand College of Anaesthetists and he is a member of the Therapeutic Assessment Group (making recommendations on pain-related drugs) for the NSW Department of Health. He has a number of the publications in the pain field and is a frequent speaker at medical meetings on pain management.

Lois Tonkin

Lois is a Senior Physiotherapist and an Associate Clinical Lecturer at the Pain Management & Research Centre at the Royal North Shore Hospital, Sydney. She has with more than 20 years specialising in pain management. She has contributed to the development of two intensive pain management programmes. She has also been actively involved in workplace rehabilitation settings where she saw the difficulties caused by poorly managed pain in injured workers. As a result of these experiences Lois has been a leading advocate of improved pain management training for physiotherapists in Australia and internationally.

Lee Beeston

Lee is a senior nurse and had specialised in pain management programmes since their inception in Australia in 1989. Lee has been working on the ADAPT pain management programme since its inception at the Royal North Shore Hospital in 1994. She completed a Masters of Science in Medicine (Pain Management) at the University of Sydney in 2001 and in 2003 she was awarded a Churchill Fellowship which enabled her to visit and study the nurse's role in pain management programmes in the UK, USA, and Canada. She performs a number of roles in the ADAPT programme, especially in patient preparation for the programme, medication reduction, and communication issues.

Practical and Positive Ways
of Adapting to Chronic Pain

MANAGE YOUR
PAIN

Revised, updated and expanded edition

DR MICHAEL NICHOLAS • DR ALLAN MOLLOY
LOIS TONKIN • LEE BEESTON

Foreword by Charles Pither FRCA

Medical Director, RealHealth Institute, London

Souvenir Press

First published by ABC Books for the
AUSTRALIAN BROADCASTING CORPORATION
GPO Box 9994, Sydney NSW 2001

First published in Great Britain in 2003 by Souvenir Press Ltd
43 Great Russell Street, London WC1B 3PD
Reprinted 2008

This revised and updated edition published 2011

Reprinted 2014, 2015, 2017

ISBN 9780285640481

Typeset by M Rules

Printed and bound in Denmark by Nørhaven

Contents

Acknowledgments

A book like this has many parents. We cannot name them all, and some might wish to remain anonymous, but we would like to especially acknowledge a number of people who have in various ways contributed to the development of this book.

First, we should thank the thousands of patients we have tried to help over the years. So much of what we know about the management of chronic pain has come from listening to their experiences. Many of them have generously agreed to participate in our research studies and almost all have completed seemingly endless questionnaires for us. It is true to say, however, that this book is an attempt to present a distillation of all that effort. We hope it will, in some way, benefit all who suffer from chronic pain.

We would also like to acknowledge a number of colleagues who have given direct assistance to us in the form of feedback on earlier drafts. Specifically, Dr Newman Harris, Associate Professor Jim Roche and Dr Ray Cook from the Royal North Shore Hospital. The remainder of the ADAPT (Active Day Patient) team have also been very forebearing in putting up with the demands the writing of this book has had on all of us. We thank them for their patience and support. We especially mention Linda Prisk for her support.

We would also like to thank Professor Michael Cousins AM, Head of the Department of Anaesthesia and Pain management at the Royal North Shore Hospital. Professor Cousins has been instrumental in the establishment of the ADAPT program at this hospital and without his vision and support the program would not have been possible.

Our spouses and families also deserve particular thanks,

especially Fiona, Moya, Bernard and Allan, who have put up with innumerable interruptions to their evenings and weekends while we huddled in front of computer screens with the latest drafts. We owe them a considerable debt.

Finally, we would like to recognise the contributions by former colleagues at the Pain Management Centre at St Thomas's Hospital in London. Specifically, Dr Charles Pither, Dr Amanda Williams, Judith Ralphs, Dr Vicky Harding and Edwina Shannon. Together with Dr Nicholas, in 1988 this group developed the original patient manual and program that form the basis of the ADAPT program. This book clearly owes a great deal to the initial manual, but we hope it also represents some of what we have learnt in the years since then. There have been many exciting developments in the field of pain over these years, but it would also be true to say that some aspects are likely to remain fixed forever.

Foreword

The journey of those who suffer from chronic pain is long and often arduous. It starts innocently enough with a problem which seems just like any other, passes through a time of bewilderment, disbelief and disillusionment; visits desolate places of loneliness, anger and self-doubt, and even then seems to have no end. Sufferers' struggling to come to terms with the reality of chronic pain know all too well the emptiest reaches of the human condition. Many such individuals talk of hitting 'rock bottom' at a time when they dare not admit to themselves that the doctors and medical systems in whom they had put such trust are apparently unable to help them. The rounds of consultations, the litany of explanations and the numerous worrisome treatments all take their toll, physically and emotionally. Sleeplessness and the side-effects of medications conspire to destroy concentration and add to the burden of fatigue. The inability to do things leads to stiffness and a decline in fitness. Inactivity leads to weight-gain which further dents fragile self-esteem. The chronic pain sufferer rightly wonders where it will all end.

How can it be, then, that I can recount hundreds of tales of people who have been down this awful road, but who have ultimately found a path out of the wasteland? Such people speak of a journey of self-discovery, which ultimately proved to be fulfilling because it provided them with an unbidden, but nevertheless ennobling, opportunity to learn more about themselves and the world in which they live. This journey has been described as the journey from patient to person, from avoidance to confrontation, from helplessness to control, from passive sufferer to active coper.

How have these voyagers managed this seemingly impossible turnaround? Have they found the miracle cure delivered by the all-knowing wise physician? Have they finally located the 'last resort' and had the winning operation? Alas! Not usually. They have, however, found their way through the desolation, by realising that the most important person on the road to recovery is the traveller him or herself. They have come to the painful recognition that if they are to get better they have to do this themselves. This realisation has not usually occurred in an instant; rather it has been a gradual awareness, like waking from a deep sleep. They have read and listened to other travellers who have made the successful journey, and perhaps been advised by those specialists in the field of chronic pain who appreciate where treatment is most fruitfully directed: giving people proper and detailed information and training in techniques to aid themselves best.

The acceptance that rescue from the all-knowing doctor is not going to occur and the dawning that they have to act themselves is perhaps the first step on the road to recovery. This is followed by the search for information about what this entails and how it is done. They ask friends and acquaintances, talk to their doctor, seek advice and surf the web. They start hearing about 'pain management' and at first find it a rather confusing notion. How can an illness that has stressed and taxed them to the ends of their sanity be managed? Besides the idea of improved management comes with the implication that up until this point in time they have been managing their problem badly. The truth is that many people do manage their pain less than optimally, but this should not imply fault or blame. If a person has never had a lesson they would not be expected to speak perfect French. They might have a few ideas but these could be improved considerably by a language course and practical instruction. It is clear that the ideas underpinning modern pain management techniques are now well proven and can dramatically alter the sufferer's life for the better. What is more they can be taught by therapists and experts who are not themselves pain sufferers. Learning pain management skills can be achieved by attending a pain management programme or seeing an individual therapist, and such treatment may be required and recommended. For many people, however, an excellent starting point is a self-help manual such as this.

There are many such books on the market and for the expectant sufferer it can be difficult to make a choice. As a pain specialist who has been preaching the merits of interdisciplinary pain management for fifteen years, I can vouch that the search for a high quality comprehensive self-help manual stops here. I say this for a number of reasons.

Dr Michael Nicholas and colleagues are respected across the world for their knowledge and understanding of chronic pain and how it can be managed effectively. They run a comprehensive and excellent programme at the University of Sydney which achieves exceptional results and incorporates many effective and usable techniques. Their research has taught us much about the reasons why chronic pain develops and how it can best be treated. They have adapted the practical knowledge gleaned from their work with many hundreds of patients and distilled it into this book. The result is not a theoretical treatise but a usable handbook moulded by the real-life problems of pain sufferers. There is nothing quirky or alternative about the ideas in this volume: they are all based on the reality of everyday life. The pain sufferer who works through it logically and follows the recommendations will be able to reduce much of the fear and uncertainty that contributes so much to the distress and despair of chronic pain. They will find tips on returning to fitness and learn about pacing techniques. They will already know how easy it is to fall into traps of negative thinking, but here they will learn more about how such situations can be perpetuated unwittingly and how they can be challenged effectively by using cognitive techniques. They will find information about using relaxation techniques and tips on how to make a gradual return to meaningful and pleasurable pastimes.

We have to be realistic and accept that books such as this are not the only treatment that pain sufferers need. Were that the case, specialists like myself who run pain clinics could shut our doors and retire. However, the basic principles and ideas set out in this book are so important that they should be part of a treatment programme offered to all chronic pain sufferers. The road may still be a tough one and there may be pitfalls and diversions along the way, but the chapters in this volume serve as both map and guidebook for the persons lost in the wastelands of chronic pain.

The message is clear – there is life after chronic pain. The path out of the wilderness starts here.

Good luck!

Charles Pither FRCA
Medical Director
RealHealth Institute
London, UK

'. . . but don't wait for the light to appear
at the end of the tunnel.
Stride down there . . .
and light the bloody thing yourself!'
S<small>ARA</small> H<small>ENDERSON</small>
Outback Sayings, Macmillan, 1996.

Introduction

Pain is something that almost everyone experiences, but what may be surprising to learn is that around 20 per cent of the population have what is called chronic or persisting pain at any one time. Chronic pain is usually described as having pain on most days for at least three months. The causes of chronic pain are many, from nonspecific back complaints to arthritis to injuries to cancer. At present, most of these conditions do not have effective or lasting cures.

Some people are affected by chronic pain more than others, but it is estimated that about 10 per cent of the population of countries such as the UK, Australia, the United States, Canada, and those of northern Europe, report that persisting pain is interfering in their daily life. In some cases the pain can be quite severe and debilitating, where people may spend most days (and nights) lying down or are very restricted in their activities. In the other 10 per cent of the population, people with persisting pain report that while they don't like being in pain, they have found ways to get around it and to get on with their lives to a reasonable extent.

This book is intended primarily for all those with chronic or persisting pain who would like to manage better than they are at present. Those who feel they are managing quite well already, may also benefit from some 'finetuning' or perhaps support for what they are already doing.

To give you an idea of whether this book could help you, try answering the questions in the checklist on page 2. On items 1 and 2, if you score 2 or less you should have something to gain from this book. On any of the items 3 to 18, if you score 2, 3 or 4, you should

Pain Self-management Checklist
M.K. Nicholas; University of Sydney Pain Management & Research Centre
Royal North Shore Hospital, 1999 ©

How often have you used these pain self-management strategies (over the last month).
Indicate your answer by circling one of the numbers (0–4) beside each item.

Thinking back over the last month, how often have you done these?

	Never	Sometimes			Very often
1. If pain stops you doing something, do you ever work out other ways to do it. (Like, if you normally sit to do a task, but find sitting is difficult due to pain, have you worked out other ways to do it? Think of an example.)	0	1	2	3	4
2. Taking regular short breaks when engaging in activities, including sitting or standing, which stir-up your pain (such as, stand up for 5 minutes every 20 minutes).	0	1	2	3	4
3. Thinking that your doctors will find a cure for your pain?	0	1	2	3	4
4. Using pain killers to allow you to do something you know will stir up your pain (like driving or standing too long, or carrying too much).	0	1	2	3	4
5. Taking more than the recommended dose of any drug related to your pain; or using alcohol for pain relief.	0	1	2	3	4
6. Taking a drug which only 'takes the edge off' your pain.	0	1	2	3	4
7. Having one or more long rest periods (more than 45 minutes) (lying or sitting) through the day (8.00 am to 8.00 pm).	0	1	2	3	4
8. Lying in bed at night worrying or getting stressed.	0	1	2	3	4
9. Due to pain, having others perform your normal household duties (like washing-up, cooking, vacuuming).					
10. Doing an activity or task until it is completed regardless of pain and then resting.	0	1	2	3	4
11. Due to pain, using aids (like sticks, braces, or collars).	0	1	2	3	4

	Never	Sometimes			Very often
12. Seeing a physiotherapist or doctor or chiropractor or other health care provider about your pain (in the last month).					
13. Thinking that increased pain means you might have injured yourself (or made your injury worse).	0	1	2	3	4
14. Thinking that doctors have missed something, or that you need more investigations to explain your pain.	0	1	2	3	4
15. Thinking that pain relief is necessary before you can become more active generally.	0	1	2	3	4
16. When your pain gets worse, do you ever have upsetting thoughts (eg, 'I can't go on; not again; why me?')	0	1	2	3	4
17. When your pain gets worse, do you ever take a tablet or have an injection?	0	1	2	3	4
18. Do you ever make comparisons between what you are like now and how you were before the onset of your pain?	0	1	2	3	4

also have something to gain from reading and learning from this book. If you don't score any 2s, 3s or 4s you probably don't need to read this book, but you might find it interesting to compare your own methods with the ones described in these pages.

If you score 3 or 4 on several of these items you should read this book closely and discuss it with your doctor. It might also help if you discussed it with a physiotherapist and a clinical psychologist with experience and training in cognitive-behavioural treatments.

If you have had this pain for more than six months to a year and no treatment seems to be helping, you should speak to your doctor about being referred to a multidisciplinary pain clinic for specialist assessment and help. Most large hospitals have a multidisciplinary pain clinic and many of these will have people who use the types of methods described in this book.

This book is based on the authors' clinical experiences in hospitals in Australia and England over the past 30 years of treating people with chronic pain. It is also based on the work and studies of clinicians and researchers from different disciplines in many countries, starting with Professor Wilbert Fordyce and colleagues from Seattle in the US in the early 1970's.

More specifically, the program described in this book has been developed by the authors at the University of Sydney Pain Management and Research Centre at the Royal North Shore Hospital in Sydney since 1994. We call our program ADAPT, as that really sums up what it's about. The ADAPT program that we run at the hospital is very intensive. Patients attend all day, Monday to Friday, for three weeks. This book is the basic manual we use. It has been revised so it can be used as a self-help book, but we recommend that it be used in conjunction with your doctor, or other health provider.

ADAPT was itself based on work done by Dr Nicholas and colleagues at St Thomas's Hospital in London, beginning in 1988. The program at St Thomas's, which we called INPUT, started out as a research project to evaluate the effectiveness of the treatment over a one-year period. Two versions of the program were compared with standard medical management of mainly just medication. The results showed that patients doing the two programs improved more than those receiving standard medical management only. Of the two versions of the program, those who attended the more intensive approach did better and this effect was still evident one year later. The more intensive version involved staying in hostel accommodation at the hospital and attending the program all day, Monday to Friday, for four weeks. The less intensive version involved patients staying at home and coming to the hospital one afternoon a week for eight weeks. Patients who attended the programs did better in terms of reduced use of medication, improved mood, improved confidence and improved activity levels. They became a lot happier and could do a lot more of their normal daily activities. They still had their pain, but it was no worse and it didn't trouble them as much as it had before.

If you are interested, an account of this study was published in the journal *Pain* in 1996 (Volume 66, pages 13–22). This journal is published by the International Association for the Study of Pain (IASP) and it is the leading international scientific journal in the field of pain.

The two main lessons we took from this study were first, the methods taught in the program are more effective than just taking medication alone, and second, the methods taught in the program are more effective if the person doing it works on them as intensively as possible.

In other words, simply doing the program in a half-hearted way is not likely to be as effective as really putting some concentrated effort into it. So, if you don't feel confident about doing this program on your own, you should ask your doctor if he or she can suggest a local clinical psychologist and physiotherapist who might be able to help. Alternatively, your closest pain management clinic might have a similar program on offer.

Although claims have been made for many different treatments for chronic pain, especially back pain, the reality is that there is no magic bullet or simple solution for chronic pain and the many problems it causes. As attractive as a quick fix would be, it is essential that all consumers of health care services remain critical of reports of breakthroughs and cures in this complex and difficult area. Almost without exception, reports in the popular media about breakthroughs in treating chronic pain have proved false. Even treatments with seemingly good scientific support do not help everyone. Equally, some people seem to benefit from almost any treatment that is devised, but that doesn't mean the treatment works for most people with the problem. Some treatments are even harmful.

This book does not claim to have all the answers, but the methods and strategies described have been supported by research in a number of countries and a list of many of these studies is provided in Appendix 1 on page 267.

Unlike a new drug or device that might be expected to 'fix' your

Overview Of ADAPT Program

The main stages of the program are outlined here.
See the individual chapters for further information on each topic.

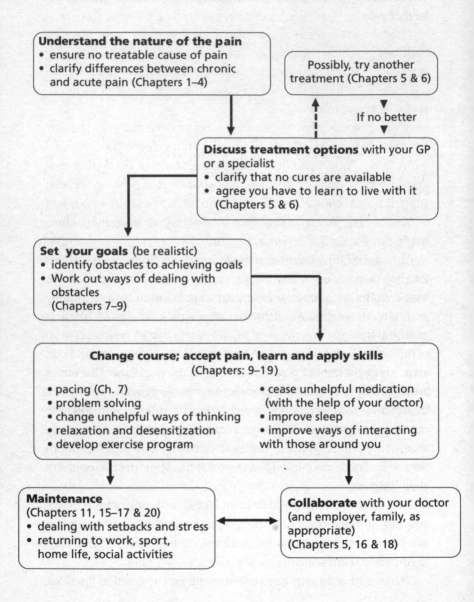

Understand the nature of the pain
- ensure no treatable cause of pain
- clarify differences between chronic and acute pain (Chapters 1–4)

Possibly, try another treatment (Chapters 5 & 6)

If no better

Discuss treatment options with your GP or a specialist
- clarify that no cures are available
- agree you have to learn to live with it (Chapters 5 & 6)

Set your goals (be realistic)
- identify obstacles to achieving goals
- Work out ways of dealing with obstacles (Chapters 7–9)

Change course; accept pain, learn and apply skills (Chapters: 9–19)

- pacing (Ch. 7)
- problem solving
- change unhelpful ways of thinking
- relaxation and desensitization
- develop exercise program

- cease unhelpful medication (with the help of your doctor)
- improve sleep
- improve ways of interacting with those around you

Maintenance (Chapters 11, 15–17 & 20)
- dealing with setbacks and stress
- returning to work, sport, home life, social activities

Collaborate with your doctor (and employer, family, as appropriate) (Chapters 5, 16 & 18)

pain for you, this book offers no instant relief. Nor does it promise total relief at some time in the future. Instead, it describes an approach to managing pain in which you, the person in pain, are expected to play an active and ongoing role. Whether it helps you achieve your goals will depend on many things. These include:

- how realistic your goals are (going parachuting may be too much to expect)
- how well you put the methods into practice (just as if you clean your teeth only once a week you wouldn't expect to have good teeth)
- how much you actually want to achieve your goals (if it would only be 'nice' but not really important, you probably won't try)
- how much support you have in your environment, at home and at work.

At different points in the book you will be asked to think about each of these issues, along with many others. The essential point is that the book is a manual. The information in the book will not change your life by itself. Only you can do that. To some extent, you have to become your own doctor/physiotherapist/psychologist. But don't despair, the book will provide guidance on all these matters.

It is our intention that the book should provide a person experiencing persisting pain with a useful guide to managing their pain themselves. We would recommend that those intending to use the book should first discuss it with their doctor, physiotherapist, chiropractor or other health care providers. If possible, it would be useful to work through the book with a health care provider acting as a sounding board. We do not want to suggest that the methods described in the book are always easy to apply, especially if you are feeling overwhelmed by your pain. If you or your doctor feel that you might need more help then it may be appropriate for you to attend a local pain management clinic where specialists in pain medicine could assess you and provide expert help.

We would also strongly recommend that you see a qualified

medical practitioner to assess your pain before you try to use the book. Your doctor may not be able to offer you any curative treatment, but he or she can certainly make sure there is nothing seriously wrong with you.

If necessary, your doctor may need to refer you to a specialist. At least you should be able to get a reasonable idea of why you have persisting pain in the first place. Clearly, if the cause is treatable, it should be treated. If there is no cure available, you will need to come to terms with having persisting pain for the forseeable future. Fruitlessly searching for a non–existent cure can end in frustration, helplessness and even despair. Not to mention the costs, to you and your family. Hopefully, you will find that this book can help you to avoid the pitfalls we all face when pain persists.

If your doctor or other health care provider disagrees with some or all of the approaches used in this book, we suggest that you discuss it with him or her. It may also be helpful to get another opinion. You could also ask your doctor if they have any better solutions and what evidence there is to support them. We strongly advise against simply accepting advice from any health care provider based only on their opinion or experience with another patient. Such opinions do not amount to good evidence in medicine these days. All health care providers have a responsibility to give you evidence to support their opinions, and that evidence should stand up to scrutiny by their peers.

The book is divided into topics. We advise you to move back and forth through different chapters as recommended in the text. Thoughtful reading and discussion, especially with other family members or good friends, can help someone suffering from persisting pain to gain new perspectives on their pain. Practising the methods outlined in this book will help you to improve your pain management skills. In turn, these improvements can result in less suffering and restoration of a more normal lifestyle despite persisting pain.

What is Chronic Pain?

1

Summary:

There are important differences between chronic and acute pain.

- Chronic pain is long-term pain and acute pain is short-term.
- Chronic pain is just as real as acute pain, but it is not due to new harm or re-injury.
- Chronic pain is maintained by changes in the central nervous system.
- At present, these changes cannot be reversed although some medications can dampen the effects for some people.
- The focus with chronic pain is managing it, not relief.
- Managing chronic pain means learning how to keep active despite the pain.
- This can also mean tackling mood and sleep problems directly instead of waiting for pain relief first.
- A co-ordinated and consistent approach to managing chronic pain is recommended. This book should help you and your carers to take a consistent approach.

It is quite likely that you and your family or friends have never really understood why your pain has gone on and on. After all, most people have pains which settle within hours or days. Without going into too much detail, it may help to briefly explain the difference between your persisting pain and the short-term pains everyone has at some time.

**Pain may be divided into two main categories:
acute and chronic**

Acute pain is short-term pain. It doesn't last very long – anything from a few seconds to a few hours or sometimes a few days or weeks. It is a type of warning signal that tells us something is wrong with our body, such as an injury. We may know what to do about it ourselves or we may go to our doctor about it. When the doctor has diagnosed what the underlying problem is, s/he will try to treat it. If the diagnosis is correct and the treatment successful the pain will be relieved fairly quickly. Sometimes acute pain will even be relieved without any medical treatment at all. An example of this would be acute back strain – in about 80% of cases this pain will ease off by itself within 2-3 weeks without any medical treat-ment (just reduced activity to begin with, followed by a gradual return to normal activities will be enough in most cases).

To re-cap, acute pain is short-lived and is normally relieved either by healing processes, some "hands on" physiotherapy or chi-ropractic treatments (where the therapist physically manipulates your muscles and joints, or applies heat or cold), some form of medical or surgical treatment, or just by taking a few simple pain killers like Paracetamol.

Chronic pain, on the other hand, is when pain persists for longer than expected. It can last for anything from 3 months to 30 or more years, despite treatment. Chronic pain is often called persisting pain and throughout this book the two terms will be used interchange-ably. There is no fixed point at which acute pain becomes chronic – it is just pain which persists longer than might be expected. Mostly, we define pain as chronic after it has been present for 3–6 months, but this varies. For example, chronic back pain often starts with short-lived episodes which settle, only to recur within a few weeks or months. Over time, these episodes may become more frequent until the pain seems to be there almost every day. However, the intensity of chronic pain usually varies and people with chronic pain often describe having good days and bad days, depending on the level of pain.

If you think you are alone in having chronic pain, we can assure you that you are not. Studies around the world have shown that between 10-20% of the population have some form of chronic pain at any one time. In countries like Australia, the US and Europe the figures are close to 20%.

Causes of pain

There are two main types of pain that may become chronic

1. Nociceptive pain

This is pain due to tissue damage like a broken bone, a sprain, or a disease like arthritis. In the case of an injury, this pain normally settles as the tissue heals, but it can persist after healing and become chronic. Sometimes the pain may settle for a period then recur and over time become almost constantly present with fluctuating severity. When you get to this stage the pain is no longer acute and nor is it being caused by the original injury. Changes will have happened in your central nervous system (your brain and spinal cord). These are explained in the next sections.

2. Neuropathic pain

Neuropathic pain is increasingly recognised as a major type of pain and is due to damage to the nerves. This can be in an arm, the spinal cord or the brain. It can often confuse doctors and other health professionals as the pain may be present in an area that has no feeling (it may be numb, but you still feel pain). The pain can also cover an unusual area, such as when it is present in the distribution of more than one nerve. Strange sensations may be reported such as electric shocks, a sensation of water flowing over the part or the area being bigger or crushed. It may also be stabbing or shooting, burning or freezing, even when the rest of you feels normal.

Neuropathic pain is best understood as being due to changes occurring in the nerves of the central nervous system (that is, the spinal cord and brain) after an injury to a nerve. The injury can be to a nerve in your arm or leg, but the effects on the central nervous system can remain long after the original injury has healed. It is still real pain even though there may be no new damage seen on scans like MRI. Some cases can be thought of as like sunburn where the skin is painful and sensitive to clothes and a hot shower. Fortunately, with sunburn the skin heals and the sensitivity goes away. But with sensitivity due to nerve damage, it may not go away, especially if changes happen in the central nervous system. Another example would be to imagine when an amplifier on a music system is turned up, in this case the same electrical signal will produce more noise. Similarly, a car alarm that is more sensitive can be set off by the wind rocking the car slightly. Your doctor may talk about this pain as being due to an increased sensitivity in your pain nerves.

Three common examples of chronic neuropathic pain are:

(1) Shingles

Shingles occurs after an infection with the chickenpox virus. Despite healing of the acute skin rash, the pain may continue in the same area for many years particularly in the elderly. They report often symptoms of the skin being sensitive and painful if touched for example with clothing or bed covers. The pain may be described as burning, stabbing and shooting. The pain can become suddenly severe with no warning and without any further injury. This is called a paroxysm. Surgical attempts have been made to cut out the pain by removing skin and deep tissue but the pain usually remains in the same site. There are a number of treatments for this and some may be successful in reducing the pain. These treatments seem to work best when they are started as soon as possible after the onset of the pain. If the pain cannot be adequately relieved then the approaches in this book should be tried to manage the pain.

(2) Phantom Limb Pain

In some situations it may be medically necessary for a foot or arm to be amputated for example to control infection or after major injury. Patients may wake up with the pain in their leg or arm and think that the operation had not been done. This is more likely if pain was present before surgery. Phantom limb pain may also be felt in the legs after spinal cord injury. Motorcyclists and water-skiers who suffer spinal cord injuries after an accident often describe this pain as crushing with electric shock sensations, as well as hot or cold sensations despite the limb usually being numb. Effective methods of reducing (but not curing) phantom limb pain are now available and these can help some (but not all) of the people with this pain. In addition, many of the coping strategies described in this book can be very helpful in managing these types of pain, but they do need a lot of practice to be effective.

(3) Complex Regional Pain Syndrome (CRPS)

This is often a very puzzling pain as it can arise in an arm or leg after an injury (like a sprained ankle or crushed hand) or no specific injury (some patients recall just bumping into something). Often there is nothing found on scans of the painful area, but yet the skin in that area can be obviously different, with swelling and colour changes being common. The person affected often reports the affected area sweats more and alternates being burning and freezing. The pain can be aggravated by even light pressure (the touch of bedsheets or a shoe, for example) and it can spread, starting in one arm and spreading to the other. This type of chronic pain can become very disabling as any movement of the affected part can make the pain worse. As a result, people with CRPS often end up avoiding the use of the affected arm (or leg) and over-using the other limb, which can then become a problem too. Some medications for neuropathic pain can help, especially if taken soon after the diagnosis is clear, but it is also very important that you start moving the affected limb as soon as possible, despite the pain. This takes courage and confidence. The methods described in this book can be very helpful in getting started and keeping going. The good news is that many of the symptoms of CRPS can be well-controlled by these methods.

Many chronic pain conditions involve both nociceptive and neuropathic elements

Many people with chronic pain have had an injury and for some reason the pain associated with that injury (or injuries) has never really gone away – or not for long – even though healing from injuries is more or less complete after about 3 months. The reason for this is not fully understood, but many scientists now believe that chronic pain is due changes in the central nervous system (that is, the spinal cord and brain) even though no actual nerve damage can be found. The main change is in the ways in which the central nervous system responds to stimulation from the rest of the body. This change is called central sensitization and we described it in the neuropathic pain section above. It is now thought that central sensistization can happen not only when a nerve is damaged (or cut, like a spinal cord injury), but also following an injury that is less specific and does not involve obvious nerve injury (like a sprain).

Putting it simply, when the central nervous system becomes sensitized it activates signals like those that follow an injury regardless of whether a new injury has happened or we have just put pressure on the skin. These signals can be interpreted by our brain as pain and we react accordingly. Unfortunately, our brain may not be able to tell the difference between a new injury and pressure on the skin. The pain you feel is still real but the cause is not due to a new injury or noxious stimulus.

However, the presence of sensitization is difficult to diagnose as it does not show up on scans. Unfortunately, even if such a process is thought to be present curative treatment options are presently limited, but we are now much more confident that these problems can be managed and their impact on our lives greatly reduced. This is the key message of this book. These processes are described more fully in Chapter 3.

Patients often want to know what type of pain they have. However, in many cases it is currently impossible to be really sure, especially if elements of both types are present. The point can also be made that if the pain can't be relieved the realistic treatment options are the same, namely, to learn to live with it.

Taking a new perspective on chronic pain

In many cases there may be no clear explanation as to why the pain is persisting. But unless you have certain diseases (such as rheumatoid arthritis), it will be true to say that chronic pain is not a warning signal of new damage. Even if you do have something like rheumatoid arthritis an increase in pain severity doesn't always mean there has been new damage. If a disease is causing your persisting pain, your doctor should be able to diagnose it and advise you on a suitable treatment. The most obvious disease of concern would be cancer. Your doctor should be able to clarify this for you. If cancer is diagnosed and appropriate treatments are undertaken good results are often obtained, especially if it is picked up early.

If you have been diagnosed with cancer and you are being treated for that you might still be experiencing continuing pain. In most cases analgesic drugs will help to ease this pain quite effectively, but you might still find the methods outlined in this book could be helpful. You would need to bear in mind that the book is mainly directed at people with non-cancer pain and so some sections may not apply to your pain. But, at the end of the day, pain is still pain, however it is caused.

Whatever the possible causes of chronic non-cancer pain, there is no way of curing these problems at present. In addition, the treatments which work for acute pain are often not helpful for chronic pain, and may even make matters worse in the long run. For example, while brief rest can help many acute pains, prolonged rest may simply make muscles and joints weaker. Long-term use of pain killers is not usually the answer either and often results in unwanted side-effects. Once physiotherapy has been adequately tried, persisting with it is unlikely to help, especially where the physiotherapist is doing things to you, like manipulation or electrical stimulation. Similarly with surgery, once it has been ruled out or tried without success, further surgery for the same chronic pain problem tends to be unsuccessful and, of course, runs more risks of making matters worse.

Once pain has become chronic (that is, lasted for more than a 3-6 months despite treatment), it is quite likely that the underlying physical problem will have become much more complicated than it was to begin with. Accordingly, a simple "cure" is most unlikely. In short, once a chronic pain problem has been thoroughly and competently investigated and treated – without success – it has to be accepted that there may be no cure for it available at present.

Whatever the original cause of your chronic pain, the persisting pain will probably have led to many changes in your daily life. For example, because of the pain you will probably do less and less of the things you did before your pain started. This will result in a loss of general fitness and strength in muscles and joints, making them stiffer. This, in turn will probably lead to more strain and pain whenever you do try to do things. For example, when their pain is more settled, many chronic pain sufferers try to catch up with all the housework or activities they haven't been able to do for a few days. This will often aggravate their pain because they have over done things. Repeatedly experiencing aggravated pain whenever you try to be active can lead to feelings of discouragement and defeat.

As a result of doing less or having to give up some of the things that were important and/or enjoyable to you (such as your job, hobbies, sport, household chores etc.) you are likely find yourself feeling more depressed, isolated, irritable or more helpless than you can remember feeling in the past.

The sense of depression and helplessness may well be aggravated by the repeated failure of different treatments to help. The ongoing pain can, of course, add to these problems, making it even harder to cope. These feelings can also lead people to become

When Chronic Pain Becomes a Problem

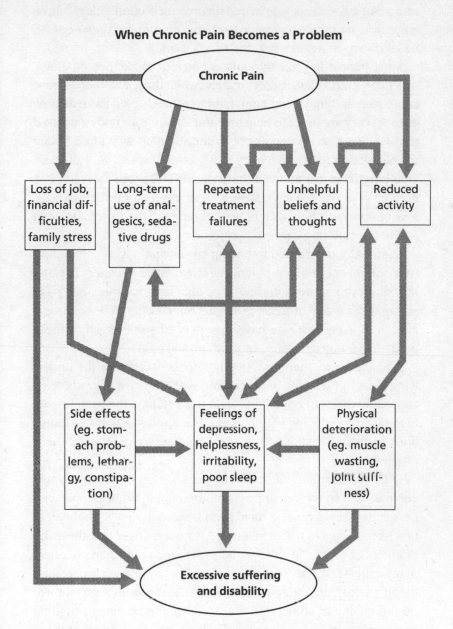

more and more desperate in their search for a cure. This is a time when you are most vulnerable to claims of miracle cures – only to be let down yet again when they don't work.

Most people in pain try various types of medicines or drugs, especially pain killers. Unfortunately, while these can help to ease acute pain and may even help at times with chronic pain, as time goes on they are likely to help less and less as your body gets used to them. Even so, many people in chronic pain will go on taking the pain killers, perhaps feeling that it is all they can do. However, with long-term use many of these tablets will probably result in a number of unwanted effects, such as an upset stomach, tiredness, loss of concentration, and bowel problems. These problems can add to the suffering caused by chronic pain.

Eventually, in addition to having chronic pain, you can end-up with a number of other problems which all have the effect of causing you even more suffering. The diagram on the next page summarises many of these problems which often follow chronic pain. It is likely that you have experienced some or all of these problems at times because of your chronic pain.

It would seem, therefore, that if there is no cure for the underlying cause of chronic pain, dealing with some of the problems caused by the pain could help to at least reduce the total impact of the pain on you and your lifestyle. The approach outlined in this book is especially aimed at helping you to deal with these problems.

Our understanding of persisting pain has become increasingly complex and so has our approach to treating it. While people with persisting pain may once have been treated mainly with medication like analgesics ("pain killers"), it is now realised that these are often not enough. This is especially true when pain starts to affect many aspects of someone's life – their home life, their work, their mood, their sleep, their recreation – all the things that go to make up the quality of someone's life. Modern approaches to treating persisting pain usually involve dealing with most or all of these areas as well as the pain. This book describes an approach that involves drawing on the expertise of medical pain specialists, clinical psychologists, physiotherapists and nurses who try to work in a collaborative way with the person in pain and their general medical practitioner.

Of course, if you can take on board the approach outlined in the book yourself, you may not need to see all of these health professionals. Working with your general practitioner on putting the program into practice may be quite enough. However, you should be prepared for quite a long struggle, with many ups and downs along the way. It can take months, or even longer, to get the hang of this approach and then you have to keep doing it.

It is important to remember, that because the pain is chronic the approach described in the book will not cure or relieve the pain. But many people have found that by dealing with the problems caused by the pain, the pain troubles them less than it once did.

Questions You May Have 2

Everyone starting this programme will have a number of questions about it. This section attempts to answer some of your likely questions. Of course, you may want to know more – or you will have other questions. If so, we suggest either reading more of the handbook or discussing your questions with your doctor or other health care providers.

1. Is the pain all in my mind?
You may have had the unfortunate experience of being told that your pain is all in your mind. At times, even you may have wondered about this.

Let us reassure you on this point. All pain is real even though no one can see it. Pain is something you feel that is as real as hunger or excitement. It is true that some people when feeling very depressed or suffering bereavement describe themselves as being in pain. But the pain this book is directed at is due to physical changes in the body, whether the changes be due to an injury, a disease or the effects of ageing.

In many cases it may not be clear why your pain has lasted so long – but that doesn't mean it is all in your mind – it is almost certainly caused by something that has gone wrong in your body. Unfortunately, there may be no cure for it at present. But what we do know is that the longer your pain goes on the more it can affect you, your daily life and your family or friends.

If there is no cure for your pain at present, a realistic alternative can be for you to try to improve the ways in which you cope with it. This does not mean that you have caused the pain in the first place.

A similar example of this is diabetes. No one would ever suggest that diabetes is "in the mind". But there is no cure for it at present and how much diabetes affects the person who has it depends largely on how well they manage it. For example, if a person with diabetes is able to maintain a suitable diet, get regular exercise and check their blood sugars daily they will maintain their health. On the other hand, if they don't do these things they may get quite sick and even hasten their death. There is little role for their doctor in this except to advise and monitor their progress. The person with chronic pain is in a similar position – although in their case poor pain management may not kill them. However, poor pain management can cause you to suffer more than you need to.

2. Will the methods described in this book stop my pain?

The pain won't go away because you cope with it better, but it should trouble you less. As you will already know, coping with pain isn't easy and there aren't any quick fixes, but if you follow the approach used in this book you should find it gets easier.

3. Is the solution simply "mind over matter"?

It's not clear what this really means, but there is unlikely to be one simple solution to all the problems caused by chronic pain. How you feel in yourself affects how you cope with your pain, but that's not mind over matter. Some people might think that all you need to overcome pain is determination or "will power". However, all the will power in the world won't help if you don't know what to do with it. It would be nice if you could just will your pain away, but as you know, it isn't possible. The methods described in this book are intended to help you find effective ways of dealing with your pain and the problems it causes you. Determination will help but you need to listen, to think and to try things out as well.

4. If my pain gets worse after exercising aren't I causing myself harm?

This is a very understandable question and will be covered fully in the physiotherapy sections of the book. But briefly, providing you do the exercises in the ways shown you should not harm yourself. In particular, you should always work within your tolerance level and try not to overdo things – even when you feel you can do more. All increases in exercise level should be carried out in a planned and steady way. If you are concerned about this issue we would encourage you to discuss it with a physiotherapist or your doctor.

In general, for people with chronic pain any extra pain after exercise will mostly be due to the effects of long-term inactivity. As your muscles and joints get fitter and stronger the extra pain and stiffness will gradually lessen. The same sort of thing happens to all of us when we try new exercises and activities after a long period of inactivity.

5. Should I give up all hope of a cure?

No. It is quite possible that either your pain will gradually lessen over time or eventually someone will find a way of treating the underlying cause and curing it. However, it is one thing to hope for an eventual 'cure' while you try to live with the pain as best you can. It is quite another thing to want to go from doctor to doctor, often repeating the same treatments and investigations, and to refuse to accept expert opinion that there is no cure possible at present.

You will find it easier to cope with your pain when you are satisfied that your pain has been investigated and treated as thoroughly and competently as possible. You will need to use your own judgement and good sense in reaching this conclusion. You will find there is a great deal you can do to help yourself by learning and practicing the approach taken in this book. At the very least, you will achieve a better quality of life.

6. If I stop the pain killers won't the pain get worse?

This is a common worry, but most people find little difference in pain overall. At the same time, most people also find they feel better in a number of ways. After you've been taking pain killers for a long period, they gradually become less helpful and you may well have tried to increase the dose or strength of your tablets. At the same time, you may have noticed a number of unwanted side-effects, such as, tiredness, stomach and bowel problems, difficulties in concentrating, and even additional aches and pains. In the end, the evidence is that pain killers offer only limited help to many people with chronic non-cancer pain and may actually worsen their situation.

The approach recommended in this book is to gradually reduce your pain killers and, at the same time, to develop other ways of coping with the pain and any withdrawal effects.

However, it is very important that you make no changes in your use of medication until you have discussed it with your doctor. We strongly advise you not to stop any drugs your doctor has prescribed for you without discussing it with him or her first. We would also recommend that if you do decide to cut back on your medication for pain that you do under your doctor's guidance.

7. I've tried everything already (without much success) so why should this programme work any better?

Of course, there are no guarantees that this programme will work any better. In the end, you can only try it and see what happens. You do have to bear in mind that this approach is not a cure, but rather a way of living with pain. It will only work if you keep practising the methods outlined in the book. In many ways, it is a bit like cleaning your teeth. If you don't clean your teeth at all, they will suffer. But cleaning them doesn't guarantee you will never have any decay, only less than you would have had if you never cleaned them.

Where you feel there are similarities between things you have tried before and the approaches described here, you may find it worthwhile thinking about why your past attempts were not successful. For example, you may well have had the right idea or intention but the problem may have been to do with the way you applied it. This is the sort of thing you could find helpful to discuss with your doctor. Perhaps it should also be pointed out that this programme is based on what has been learned from people with chronic pain – in this country and elsewhere – over a long period. In other words, there is a great deal of evidence that it can help – providing you put it into practice and keep doing it.

8. It sounds good in theory, but will it work for me?

One thing we can assure you, is that success with this programme does not depend on the severity of your pain, the site of your pain, the original cause of your pain, or how long you have had it.

We don't expect you to believe in this approach before you have tried it. However, we have found that most of the people who have gone through the programme have got something out of it and many have made major changes because of it. How much someone gets out of it depends on a number of things, such as:

- **how much you put into it** (if you don't try the techniques and methods covered in the programme you won't get much out of them – thinking and talking about your pain won't be enough);
- **how ready you are for it** (if you don't accept that your doctors have done all that is possible, you may not be ready);
- **other worries or pressures** (stresses at home or financial worries may make it harder for you to focus on the programme).

9. Is this the right treatment for me?

Many of the people who attend our programme feel that they are different from other patients – either because their pain is in a different place or the cause is different. As a result, they feel that while the programme is the right approach for some people, it is not the right one for them.

To some extent, this could suggest they haven't come to terms with the chronic nature of their pain. Whatever the differences between people with chronic pain, there are also many similarities. For example, most of the people attending our programme would agree that their pain has disrupted their lives in many ways. Whatever the cause or site of their pain, all of the people coming to this programme have a pain problem that is not curable at present. All have to learn to live with their persisting pain.

The results achieved so far by patients attending the programme (and other similar programmes) show that all people with chronic pain can benefit from the programme, regardless of their differences.

10. Am I too old (or young) for this approach?

This concern has much in common with some of those already covered. But if you have persisting pain and you would like to manage it better than you are at present then it doesn't matter how old you are. If you are older you might not be able to do as much as some other people, but that would apply whether you had pain or not. It is also our experience that there are more concerns about using medication for pain in both the young and the elderly.

Everyone using this book should try to apply the methods described to themselves as much as possible.

11. Is the ADAPT approach suitable for people with pain due to cancer?

Yes. Providing your cancer is being addressed medically as much as possible (usually with some combination of medications, radiation or surgery), it can still be helpful for you to play a role in managing your pain. The methods outlined in the book can be useful regardless of the cause of pain. In the case of pain due to cancer, the ADAPT methods should be seen as an adjunct to the normal medical treatments for cancer and associated pain. The ADAPT methods can still help to improve your quality of life and may help you to reduce your reliance on analgesics (pain killers) as the only means of controlling your pain.

12. What about people with pain due to HIV/AIDS?

Yes. The answer would be the same as for those with pain due to cancer. The cause of pain is not so relevant when it comes to self-management principles. In fact, most of the principles outlined in this book are useful for the management of all chronic illnesses. They are not intended as cures, but rather to help the person live as well as possible with the illness.

13. What about people with spinal cord injury pain?

As more than half of people with spinal cord injuries report chronic pain associated with their injuries pain self-management is a major challenge on top of all the other adjustments they have to make. For several years now we, and several of our colleagues, have been testing these methods with people who have spinal cord injury pain and were referred by their doctors to our clinic. We have found that these methods can help this group, but as with everyone else, you have to do them regularly for several weeks before you will see benefits. Also, like everyone with chronic pain, you will need to keep practising these strategies as long as your pain persists. Naturally, there are some differences between those with spinal cord injuries and other people with chronic pain that are important to keep in mind when applying the methods described in this book.

The most obvious difference is that many of the exercises described here are not possible for people with spinal cord injuries. However, the principles of trying to keep as active as possible, doing whatever exercises are possible, using pacing, remain important.

The more psychological strategies, however, are just as applicable regardless of whether or not you have a spinal cord injury. The chapters on dealing with unhelpful thoughts, emotional distress, setting goals, developing an activity upgrading plan, sleep management, and using strategies like relaxation and focusing on the pain are especially important.

What's Going On In Your Body When Pain Is Chronic?

Pain is experienced by people of all ages. However some people are born unable to feel pain. This may seem wonderful but these individuals may injure themselves without knowing it, as they don't have pain to act as a warning system. Pain can be a very useful warning signal and can protect us from serious harm. But this really only applies to acute pain. Chronic pain doesn't seem to have any useful purpose. By the time pain becomes chronic it is no longer acting as a warning signal. You've had it investigated so you either know what has caused it or you've been told you don't have a serious injury or disease. But it can still be a mystery. Why isn't it going away?

If you are confused about the basis of your pain or if you feel the doctors must have missed something, it can be difficult to accept ongoing pain. You may wonder if you do try to get on with your life, despite your pain, could you risk making things worse. This could leave you feeling unsure about what to do or where to go.

For these reasons it is important to learn a little about what can be going on in your body when pain persists even though you've had expert investigations and treatment. This will help you to understand the approach that is used in this book. This approach requires you to accept that you have ongoing pain but you are OK.

Summary

At any one time about 1 in 5 people experience some form of chronic pain, but the causes can differ between people. It often starts with an injury (like a broken bone) or an illness or disease (like Arthritis), but sometimes there is no clear reason. For example, with chronic low back pain a specific cause is often difficult to find. In many people the site of their pain may not be where the trouble lies, even though it feels like it. So, cutting off your arm may not fix the problem of chronic arm pain. In fact it could make matters worse.

As we mentioned in Chapter 1, recent research has shown that when we experience pain over a long time changes can develop in nerves in the spinal cord and the brain (the part called the central nervous system). These changes may not be seen on a scan but they can make us feel pain even when we seem to do nothing harmful. We call this a sensitization effect.

A common example of a sensitization effect is sunburn. When you have a shower with sunburned skin it seems to burn or sting. We know the effect is due to the sunburn not the hot water. When the sunburn settles the shower water stops stinging. This type of sensitization of your skin is called 'peripheral sensitization' and it is reversible with no lasting effects. Unfortunately, when the nerves in your spinal cord get sensitized it is not so reversible. This is called 'central sensitization' because it occurs in your central nervous system.

The key feature of central sensitization is feeling more pain when we do something that shouldn't be painful, like a slight bump or just a handshake. Your doctor might call this 'allodynia'. But if a mildly painful stimulus is felt as very painful your doctor might call that 'hyperalgesia'. In both cases, the pain will seem quite out of proportion to the incident that triggers it. This can make you think there must be something seriously wrong and that you should avoid that activity in future. You might also worry that if you tell others about your experience they might think you're imagining things or exaggerating. But, you're not – these are common characteristics of chronic pain conditions.

There are two main types of pain. Nociceptive pain follows an injury to our skin, muscles, bones or tendons. This pain usually settles with healing, but not always. If it becomes chronic then it may come to involve changes in our nerves, like central sensitization. At this stage such pain is much harder to treat successfully.

Neuropathic pain is pain due to nerve damage. Central sensitization effects are a common feature of neuropathic pain and they are often long-lasting. These sensitization effects can also be experienced even when no nerve damage is found. In some cases this might be because nerve damage can be difficult to find, but in other cases it might be a more subtle effect of changes in our nervous system that we don't yet fully understand.

Regardless of how chronic pain starts, all pain involves a chain of events in your nervous system, with one thing leading to another. The final stage of this chain of events is the pain you feel. Before that moment, pain is really just a lot of activity or signals in

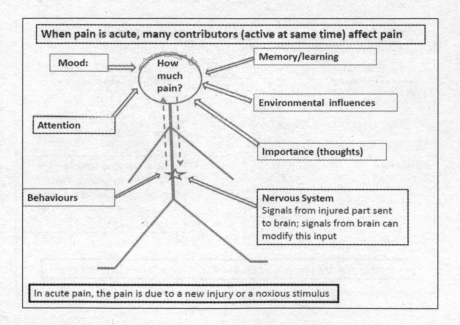

When pain is acute, many contributors (active at same time) affect pain

Mood:

How much pain?

Memory/learning

Environmental influences

Attention

Importance (thoughts)

Behaviours

Nervous System
Signals from injured part sent to brain; signals from brain can modify this input

In acute pain, the pain is due to a new injury or a noxious stimulus your nervous system. It is your brain's job to make sense of this activity and interpret the signals as 'pain'. Some of this 'brain work' will be outside your awareness, but some will be more conscious, especially if you can stop and reflect on it.

What your pain ends up feeling like depends not just on nerve signals coming up your spinal cord to your brain, but also on how you view the experience. If you see it as threatening you are likely to experience it as more severe and disturbing. But if you see it as something understandable and not threatening then it will seem less severe or disturbing. The diagrams in the boxes provide a sim-plified demonstration of what happens in your body when you have acute pain, using a lower back pain as an example, and what happens when the pain becomes chronic.

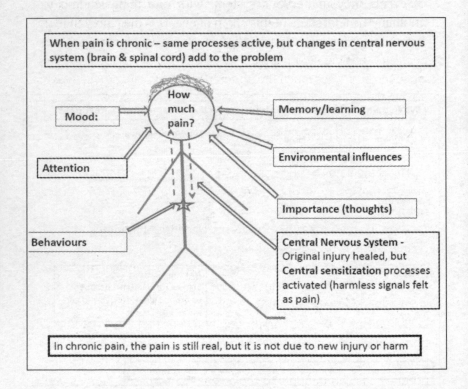

When the pain becomes chronic these contributors are repeated over months or years. It is easy to see how they can become learnt responses that occur almost automatically.

In the next sections we briefly describe the chain of events that can lead to the development to chronic pain like you have been experiencing.

Nervous system

1. From skin to spinal cord

Damage to our skin (like a cut or burn) or a sprain (like a sprained ankle) turns on small sensors close to the surface of the skin or tendons or muscles. These sensors are called nociceptors (related to the term "noxious", meaning harmful). This is the first stage in the experience of pain. The nociceptors are linked to nerves end in the spinal cord (inside the spine). The messages (which are in the form of electrical signals) travel from the nociceptors, along the nerves to the spinal cord which sends them to the brain. It is only when the messages reach the brain that we feel pain, providing we are awake or conscious.

In many ways this is like what happens in a telephone system, where electrical messages travel along telephone wires until they are converted to sound in the handset.

This can happen very quickly. To give you an idea of how quickly, think of how quickly you can pull your hand away from a hot pan.

Soon after an injury the tissues around the injury site start to change. This is part of the healing process. We notice things like swelling, some redness in the skin, as well as pain and the area can also feeling hotter. These effects are due to tiny gaps in the small blood vessels widening to allow through part of the blood called plasma that is rich in protein and cells that can fight infection. Next, specialised cells begin to lay down a very strong material called collagen to form scar tissue. In many tissues the normal cells can multiply to replace damaged tissue. Nerves can regrow as well, but unfortunately the spinal cord cannot. Recovery of sensation depends on the nerves regrowing down the correct tunnel or sheath.

As healing proceeds, the messages that signal pain gradually settle and so does the experience of pain. Even after major surgery, most people do not require much pain relief medication after 3-4 days. Patients are encouraged to get moving as soon as possible as this helps to reduce complications and to promote recovery.

2. Spinal cord and brain stem

The spinal cord also plays a key role in the experience of pain. The spinal cord is a collection of specialised nerves and cells that lie within the spine. There are connections with the nerves that carry information to and from different parts of our body. The spinal cord is like a complicated telephone exchange, handling information coming in from nerves all through our body. The messages from these nerves are then sent up the spinal cord to the brain. At the base of the skull the spinal cord is connected to an area we call the brain stem which is the lower part of the brain. The brain stem plays a role as a filter, deciding which messages are passed on to the brain.

Not all pain messages reach the brain. They all reach the spinal cord but their entry to the brain can be blocked. In 1965 two scientists, a Canadian called Professor Ronald Melzack and an Englishman called Professor Patrick Wall suggested that there was a type of gate within the spinal cord which allowed messages to pass through to the brain only if it was open. But if the gate is closed the pain messages wouldn't get through. This gate can be opened or closed by other nerve messages. It is important to understand that this theory mainly applied to acute pain, not chronic pain. Since 1965 our understanding of the nerve processes underlying acute and chronic pain has developed enormously, but the basic ideas outlined in 1965 remain relevant, especially for acute pain.

It has been known for time that the gate in the spinal cord can be closed by nerve signals indicating pressure or heat. So, rubbing a painful area when you are injured can ease the pain you feel. Putting a hot or cold pack on the painful area can also help. These measures don't fix the injury but they can block the pain signals for a short period. TENS machines and acupuncture may work the same way (see Chapter 6).

The gate can also be closed by messages coming down from the brain. So, if you can distract your attention from the pain, or if you are not distressed about the pain, you won't feel it as much. In an emergency situation, like a car accident, you can be injured but not realize it because your brain is too busy dealing with practical tasks like getting out of the car. You may only notice the pain when you are starting to relax and realize you are still alive. All these examples indicate the gate, or modulation system, is working to limit the pain you feel. This allows you time to deal with an emergency before you have to deal with any injuries. This mechanism has probably helped all animals, including humans, to survive as long as we have.

Examples of this gating system are often reported by people injured while playing heavy contact, physical sports but not noticing the pain until the game is over. Similarly, many soldiers who have been injured in battle have reported feeling little pain until later. Unfortunately, it doesn't seem possible to keep the gating mechanisms closed forever. So this mechanism mainly applies to acute pain.

Just as the gate can be closed by messages from the brain, it can also be opened by the brain. If, for example, you focus your attention on the pain and worry about what it might mean, the gate can be opened allowing more nociceptive signals through and you will feel more pain. This can also happen without any conscious awareness on your part.

In our research, for example, we have found that even saying things like "this is terrible", "I can't cope with this", or "I can't go on" can lead to pain being more severe and troubling. If you're not sure about this, try a short experiment. Hold a few blocks of ice in your hand (with fingers closed around them) for about 2 minutes while you say these sorts of statements to yourself and see what happens to the pain. Put the ice down, dry and rest your hand for a few minutes then repeat the exercise, but this time try saying things like "this is just ice", "I know I'm OK", and "I'll just observe the sensation for a couple of minutes and see what happens".

Compare the two situations – one where you are saying alarming things to yourself about the sensation, the other when you are more neutral and not alarmed, just curious. In both situations the noxious stimulus (the ice) is the same. The only difference is what you are saying to yourself about it. We call the alarmist thoughts 'catastrophising' and have found that when people think about their pain in a catastrophic way it hurts more and distresses them more. This means the experience of pain is not all due to the injury. It's meaning to you also influences how it feels.

When pain becomes chronic the gating mechanism described by Melzack and Wall doesn't apply as much because the original injury and source of the nociceptive signals has healed. Instead we have to look at other mechanisms in the central nervous system, especially the brain, to understand chronic pain.

3. The brain
The brain stem passes the pain messages up to an area of the brain known as the cerebral hemispheres or forebrain. This is the part of the brain that deals with thoughts, memories and emotions. It is only when this part of the brain has had a chance to make sense of the pain signals that we feel the pain that we know.

The brain tries to work out what the pain means to us. Which part of our body is it coming from? Should we worry about it or is it just a minor irritation to be ignored? Is it like something we've had before? What should we do about it? All these questions can happen in an instant and you may only be aware of them if you sit down and try to think them through later. The end result is that we can be acting on the pain signals even before we've really considered the best option to take. It can be as if we are on 'automatic pilot'. In the case of acute pain that can be helpful. So the rapid response helps if your hand touches a hot pan and you need to withdraw it before it is badly burned. But if the pain is chronic and we are not in danger of being harmed the immediate response to an increase in pain may not be the best option.

In the case of chronic pain the pain signals are not a warning of new damage. Instead, they may be just normal sensations of pressure or strain that are misinterpreted by the brain as being a warning signal, like acute pain. This is the sensitization and amplification effect mentioned earlier. Remember the example of sunburned skin – the stinging pain we feel under the shower is not due to new damage. Instead the normal temperature shower water is felt as if it is much hotter than it is, because our sensitized skin amplifies the signals.

In the case of major damage to nerves, such as when a foot is amputated or the spinal cord is severed, no nerve signals can get through to the brain from below the site of the damage. But at least half of those people with these injuries report ongoing pain from below that point. We might call this 'phantom pain', but to the person with the pain it is not a phantom. In fact, this is an example of the brain responding to the signals it is receiving (and not receiving) from the spinal cord. This is an example of neuropathic pain, where there is clear nerve damage.

In these types of neuropathic pain there is often a mix of sensitization effects as well as the effects of the absence of expected nerve signals from below the injury site. It is as if the brain interprets not getting the normal signals from below the level of the injury as pain and other unpleasant sensations (such as itch and 'ants crawling under the skin'). These other sensations can also be unpleasant even if not painful. They are examples of what is called "dysaesthesia".

The longer we experience chronic pain the more these effects are repeated. It is not difficult to imagine a possible consequence of these repeated effects is that our responses to these repeated pain signals become learnt, like a habit. Like a habit they can be triggered by cues or reminders, often quite spontaneously. Just like a tune we haven't heard for a while can stir dormant feelings in us. In the case of pain, a famous ballerina once reported that she just had to hear the music from one of her favorite dances to feel the pain she used to get from dancing on her toes. Similarly, some people with chronic pain report their pain can be stirred up even by seeing others obviously in pain. This is known as an empathy response.

If your brain is doing all this you might wonder why you can't just block the pain out mentally and stop it. Unfortunately, no one seems able to do this very well or not for very long. But these observations about pain mechanisms do offer some clues for ways we might be able to combat chronic pain through our brain.

A key finding of recent research is that if your brain is receiving normal sensations from activities such as walking, exercising, swimming, and moving as normally as possible (that is, not too cautiously) then the pain responses in your brain can be reduced and the pain will trouble you less. This is especially true if you can accept the pain and stop fighting it or worrying about it (that is, not catastrophising). In general, leading as normal a life as possible and making the most of life can help to keep pain manageable and minimise its impact.

Another reason for resuming normal activities despite your pain is that it can help to disconfirm expectations and fears that something awful might happen. When you find you can do these things again and enjoy them, the pain will also trouble you less.

As you might have found with the ice experiment the significance of the pain (or what it means to you) can influence what you experience. If you can accept that the pain signals are not threatening and you are OK, you will experience them quite differently. They are just sensations, like background noise. On the other hand, if you repeatedly react to chronic pain as if it is acute (and a sign of new injury) you can remain in a state of distress which can make the pain feel even worse and more distressing.

You may not even be aware that these processes are playing such a major part in your experience of pain. Over time, these response patterns can become almost automatic, but you can become aware of the patterns and your responses. A cake once mixed and baked is very different to the individual ingredients from which it was made. Just as you can't separate the ingredients of a cake so it may be difficult to separate the pain from your emotions, memories, thoughts, and beliefs. But understanding what is going on in your nervous system and realizing that chronic pain is not a threat to your body can help the process of accepting it and getting on with your life again.

4. Autonomic nervous system

This is a part of the nervous system over which we normally have little control but we can learn to influence it. It is made up of two parts: the sympathetic and the parasympathetic nervous systems. The sympathetic part controls our "flight and fight" reaction. If we are frightened and need to prepare ourselves for something that we think is dangerous the sympathetic nervous system causes changes like an increase in our heart rate and increased blood flow to the muscles. We also become more alert so that we can react quickly. The parasympathetic nervous system has the opposite effect – it slows us down.

Unfortunately, sympathetic hyperactivity (that is, over-activity) can occur even if there is no real threat. Being afraid of mice, harmless spiders or open spaces are common examples. The heart will race, sweating may occur and a feeling of anxiety is present. It may even lead to a panic attack. Pain can also produce this response which can be very distressing. Fortunately if the pain cannot be relieved, we can learn to control this response which should reduce any distress.

The sympathetic nervous system can also become hyperactive in a condition called reflex sympathetic dystrophy or complex regional pain syndrome. This usually follows nerve injury, but the nerve injury can be very minor in some cases. For example a hand or foot will become painful, stiff, sweaty and change in colour and appearance. As with other pain conditions there are a number of medical treatments that may help. But they are often not enough to resolve it completely and the approaches in this book should be included in the treatment plan.

5. Bones and the spine

Humans have an internal skeleton consisting of a backbone or vertebral column which is connected by specialised joints to the head, the arms and the legs. These bones and joints grow with the person. They provide remarkable flexibility and the capacity for a range of complex movements through the attachment of muscles, tendons and ligaments across the joints. Being upright, humans experience significant pressures on the bony skeleton. Movement adds to these stresses through the contraction of muscles anchored to the skeleton.

The anatomy of the spine

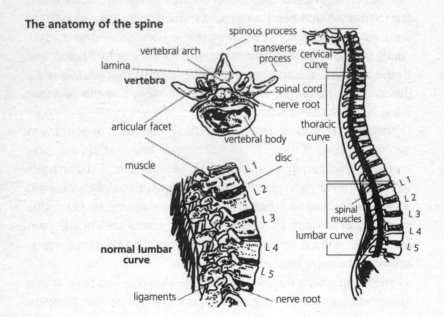

spinous process
vertebral arch
transverse process
cervical curve
lamina
vertebra
spinal cord
nerve root
articular facet
thoracic curve
vertebral body
muscle
disc
L 1
L 2
spinal muscles
L 3
normal lumbar curve
L 4
lumbar curve
L 5
ligaments
nerve root
L 1
L 2
L 3
L 4
L 5

Within the protection of the backbone lies the spinal cord. This is linked to the brain through the base of the skull and to the body by nerves which pass through spaces between the bones which make up the spine. Messages travel to and from the brain to trigger sensation and activate muscles respectively as described above.

In this disposable consumer age we don't expect things to last very long yet we expect the human body to last a lifetime, possibly at least 70-80 years. What makes it all possible is the human body's ability to repair and regenerate itself. This is usually a slow process unless trauma occurs and then the body rapidly repairs itself.

As we get older the supple **discs** between the vertebrae (the bones of the back) become more rigid and fibrous, lose height and lead to restrictions in the amount of cushioning and movement.

Also with age the effects of wear and tear or **spondylosis** become apparent with thickening of the surface of the vertebrae and new irregular bone laid down around the edge of the discs. The lower lumbar vertebrae are affected most. This adds to the limitation of movement caused by changes in the discs and arthritis of the paired facet joints (see glossary) may also contribute. These changes start from about 30 years of age and progress at different rates depending on the individual. At the age of 60 years, wear and tear is evident on most x-rays. Calling these changes "abnormal" is wrong as they are clearly "normal" for that age group.

Surprisingly there is no clear relationship between the changes seen and pain experienced. An individual may have advanced degeneration of the spine yet experience little or no pain yet a younger person with a normal looking x-ray may have severe pain. A mistake is easily made here. Saying that backache is due to spondylosis may result in other important causes being missed. It is important that you don't try to deal with "wear and tear" effects by avoiding activities. In general, keeping fit and active keeps us supple and healthy.

Vertebral slips. The bones of the vertebral column are held in position like the mast of a ship with muscles and ligaments acting like ropes. The articulations of the facet joints also provide stability. But as a result of wear and tear of the joints or if a break occurs in the bony arch at the back of the vertebra, it can slip forward, which is called a spondylolisthesis. This is present in 1.5% of the Australian population but is usually painless. A slip in the other direction is called a retrolisthesis. As this slip in the vertebrae can stretch the nerve roots pain in the legs may occur.

Narrowing of the vertebral canal: The canal inside the backbone in which the spinal cord lies varies in size in different individuals. In about 15% of the population the canal is tight, a condition known as spinal stenosis. It may have just developed that way or there may have been degeneration of the facet joints and discs that lead to ingrowths into the bony canal. The usual symptoms are numbness and pain in the back and legs on walking. This is eased by sitting and usually by bending forward as this seems to allow more space in the bony canal.

Joints: Each bone in the body is connected to at least one other. At this junction there is a joint of some type. There are many types of joint, for example the hip is a ball and socket joint whilst the ankle and knee are like hinge joints. The inner surface of the joint is lined by very slippery material to minimise resistance to movement.

Wear and tear can occur in these joints. This is known as osteoarthritis. Heavily-used joints, such as hips, knees, and the joints in the spine, develop roughened surfaces and in an attempt to repair this the body lays down new tissue. Around the edges of the joint bone is laid down. This can effectively splint the joint, restricting its movement. At the same time, within the joint an inflamatory process occurs. This makes the joint tender and can be painful. Over time, this pain may spread to surrounding areas. This is called referred pain. So, wear and tear of a hip may be experienced as pain in the knee.

Muscle: There are different types of muscle in the body. There is skeletal muscle which is the "red" muscle and smooth muscle which occurs in the lungs and bowel. The heart also has a special type of muscle. Skeletal muscle usually spans a joint. By contracting, movement of a joint will occur. Most muscles have an opponent, a muscle that will counteract the effect by having an opposite action across a joint. Unfortunately muscles will weaken if not used and lose their bulk. They can also shorten and in doing so limit the movement of a joint. When you try to use muscles in this state they tend to be painful for a period. Anyone who does unaccustomed exercise will be familiar with this phenomenon. Fortunately, with ongoing use, the muscles can recover and this pain lessens.

In certain conditions, however, there may be taught bands within the muscle, which may respond to stretching, but not totally. As a result some pain may persist. This is known as myofascial pain if it is localised to one area. If it is widespread it may be classified as fibromyalgia by some doctors.

Ligaments: Ligaments play an important role in support and therefore the movement of joints. There are two types of ligament. Most ligaments in the body are made from white fibrous tissue which is usually non-elastic and unstretchable. It will stretch but only after prolonged strain. There is another type of ligament that is elastic and will return to it usual length after stretching. This type is present between the bones of the back allowing the spine to bend. Stretch exercises can assist this process.

In summary, many structures in the body can contribute to chronic pain, either as a cause or a reaction to the effects of pain, especially disuse. None of these structural changes can fully account for what people with chronic pain actually experience. Many of the bodily changes with chronic pain are not structural but functional. That is, processes like central nervous system sensitization change the ways our nervous system functions. In this case, making the nervous system more sensitive. These functional changes can explain how normally harmless activities or stimuli can be experienced as pain. These functional changes cannot be seen on scans, but scans can rule out major structural damage. Some of these changes are modifiable, but not always completely. The options for treatment for chronic pain conditions will be addressed in the following chapters.

What X-rays, CT and MRI Scans Tell Us

The word 'imaging' is a term used to describe tests that provide pictures or scans of parts of the body. As these tests have become more advanced they have allowed us to look inside the body without the need for an operation. Where the cause of pain might once have been put down to a condition such as 'lumbago' or a 'strain', new tests are helping doctors to work out exactly what is wrong. Scans are particularly helpful in excluding worrying conditions such as cancer and infections.

The scans have to be interpreted very carefully by experts taking into account the problem that the patient has. Because the techniques are very sensitive, findings on the scan that seem to be abnormal and of concern may in fact be normal for that person or a person's age group. This is particularly true as we get older and wear and tear inevitably occurs. Even in the younger age group a disc bulge may be found on a scan of a person with back pain and it might be assumed that this was the cause of the pain. Recent scientific studies have found similar disc bulges in people without pain, however. Also, conditions where the disc is damaged such as an internal disc disruption or an annular tear, are often painful but are also seen on scans in people who are not reporting pain. Damage to intervertebral discs can certainly be the cause of back pain but this diagnosis has to be made with caution before treatment is recommended.

It is important to remember that scans do not show pain. At one extreme a person may have severe degeneration (wear and tear) of the spine that shows up on an X-ray but no pain, while someone who is very disabled by back pain may have little to find on any tests.

> Geoff was a senior radiologist and had worked as a hospital specialist for many years. To liven up a teaching session with a group of doctors, he had an MRI scan performed on himself and presented this to the audience. He made up a history of someone who was unable to work because of pain. The scan showed marked wear and tear and surgery was considered an option. The surgeons were very surprised when Geoff told them the scan was of his back and that although he had some pain he worked long hours and was physically active in his garden at the weekends.

Scans are important but provide only part of the picture. It is necessary first of all to assess the person and their problem by talking to the person, finding out about the nature of their problem, how it started and then undertaking a thorough examination.

Accepting negative scans in a positive way

Scans play an important part in trying to pinpoint where the pain is coming from but often no abnormality shows up. This can be a very disappointing result as both you and your doctor know that to cure the pain you need to know what is causing it. The doctor may present the scan as being negative and apologise for that by saying, 'I am sorry that the scans are negative, I cannot find where the pain is coming from'.

A more helpful way of looking at it, however, is to think of the scans as 'positive' if they do not show any abnormality. That means that you should be reassured that you are okay and that you are unlikely to have a serious problem such as a fracture, an infection or cancer.

It is true that doctors are getting better at identifying the cause of the pain but the cause of every pain that people experience is not yet known. For example, in many cases of back pain, doctors can't be sure where the pain is coming from. And although the doctor may be absolutely sure where the pain is coming from, there is no certainty that this pain can be fixed.

Current imaging techniques

X-rays

The discovery of X-rays and their use in medicine was a significant breakthrough. X-rays are absorbed by different parts of the body and produce 'shadows' on the film. Bone absorbs X-rays and appears white on the film, whereas soft tissue appear dark. Fractures are most frequently diagnosed with X-rays but they do not help with seeing detail such as a disc pressing on a nerve or on the spinal cord. And X-rays do not show pain.

CT scans

For this type of scan the patient is placed in the CT (computerised axial tomography) tube. X-rays are passed through the body and picked up on the other side. The way in which the X-rays have been 'changed' by the body is fed into a computer that makes a series of complex calculations. The result is a picture of the body in cross-section. Bony problems in particular are sensitive to this technique.

MRI scans

The MRI (magnetic resonance imaging) scanner consists of a large magnet. This interacts with particular properties of your body to produce signals that are processed by a computer to form detailed images. The scanner allows us to look inside any part of the body. It is particularly useful for 'seeing' the spinal cord and nerve roots, without having to operate. The technique also provides an idea of the chemical make-up of the disc and allows us to recognise conditions like disc degeneration at an early stage. A clear advantage over CT scanning is that as X-rays are not used there is no risk from radiation.

Bone scans

In this type of scan tiny amounts of radioactive material are injected into the body. Areas where there is damaged tissue, an injury or an infection accumulate more of the material and can be detected by a special scanner. This is a very sensitive method of pinpointing problem areas. At times, these scans will reveal things that don't show up with other methods. They are not always necessary, however, and their use must be governed by the clinical judgment of your doctor.

Myelography

This refers to the injection of a special dye into the fluid around the spinal cord. The dye enables the structures inside the spinal canal to be seen on an X-ray or CT scanner. This test does carry some risks and in many ways it has been replaced by the advent of MRIs.

Working with **5** Your Doctor

When your doctor was a medical student, pain management as we know it today, was probably not taught in great depth. There have been many changes since then, including more availability of specialised training and recognition of the need for multidisciplinary teams to help with the complex problems of people with chronic pain. A typical 'team' in a hospital pain clinic would be a medical specialist, a clinical psychologist or psychiatrist, a physiotherapist and a nurse. Other health professionals, such as social workers, occupational therapists and dietitians, may contribute as well. For best results, a hospital team should work closely with your family doctor as he or she is the health care provider who is closest to you and will be able to provide ongoing and readily available help.

Not all people with chronic pain need to see a multidisciplinary team at a hospital, but they are available if your doctor thinks it might help for you to see them. However, even the people who have attended our ADAPT program, which is in a hospital, are strongly encouraged to maintain close links with their doctor in the future, for as long as their pain persists.

It is important to establish a good 'working' relationship with your family doctor. This is particularly so when you have to manage a chronic problem for which there is no cure, such as diabetes, heart disease, asthma or chronic pain. For chronic pain, it is important that the individual continues to function and manage the pain in the best way possible, and this requires an active approach. Instruction is needed on how to best manage persisting pain. Most family doctors encourage activity despite pain (unless there is a good reason to rest), and sensible use of pain killers. Through their experience and training they will recognise those who are doing well and those who need more help than they can provide. If you are not doing as well as you would like or should be, then you are likely to benefit from the help of a multidisciplinary team.

Getting the best from your family doctor

Keep in regular contact with your doctor

It is best to think of the family doctor as your doctor, with all other health professionals providing specialist opinions and treatment. Your family doctor is not a mind reader, so you will need to be clear about your pain. They can't know what you don't tell them. Keep your doctor informed of any changes in your pain or function and make sure that you ask for regular reports from other health professionals to be sent to your doctor. If you see a new doctor, make sure that you tell your family doctor. If you feel that you are not making enough progress then discuss getting a second opinion.

See your doctor on good days too

Avoid just attending your doctor when you are in more pain or really distressed. This unfortunately only allows the doctor to manage the crisis that they are presented with. By seeing your doctor on good days other areas can be explored with you without pain and distress being such a major factor. A major crisis should be followed by an appointment to try to work out why it occurred and how best to manage such a situation in the future. Often a crisis is brought on by things such as poor planning, not pacing activities, unhelpful thoughts and lack of use of stress management skills. These are all things that you need to do. Nobody else can do them for you.

Make notes before you go to the doctor

Write down any questions you would like to ask your doctor as they come to mind. This is helpful for your doctor too. If you don't, you are likely to forget something that has been bothering you. Remember, your doctor has many patients and if you don't ask something he or she might assume that you know all about it.

Remember that your doctor is human

There are only certain things that your doctor can do to relieve your pain. 'Quick fixes' are rare. You may feel that your doctor is not doing very much, when in fact your doctor may be waiting for the natural history to take its course and for you to get better. Your doctor will try to help as much as possible, but you must also look at what you are doing to manage your problem as well. Try to work with your doctor on these problems rather than expecting your doctor to have all the answers and that it is their responsibility to fix the problem for you.

Be honest

Sometimes when people are distressed by pain they will do things that are not in their best interests long term. For example, they may take more than the recommended dose of a drug or even take drugs that have been prescribed for a family member or friend. Your doctor needs to know about this so that they can help you.

Be realistic

There are only certain treatments for persisting pain, and many of them have only a small success rate. Very few are likely to totally relieve pain, although new treatments are becoming available all the time. Remember, all drugs have side effects.

Look at your own pain management

There are a number of things that you can do to manage your pain. This is called active pain management and is, of course, the subject of this book. Let your doctor know about your achievements in managing your pain. Try not to focus solely on the problems and failures. Recognise your achievements too.

Feel confident to reject a treatment

You may need to work out ways of saying no to offers of medication or treatment that you are not interested in. Your doctor will be pleased to see you taking more responsibility for managing your pain, since doing so also lifts some of the burden off their shoulders. This can help in making your relationship a more equal, collaborative one, rather than a one-sided arrangement where the doctor feels everything is up to him or her to solve.

Questions to ask your surgeon

If you are considering surgery, it is very important that you find time to discuss the risks and benefits of surgery with your surgeon well before you are admitted to hospital. Avoid, if possible, having these discussions the night before your operation. Most surgeons will try to answer your questions but remember that they may not have all the answers as the full picture may not be available. Research is constantly taking place so more answers will become available over time.

Clearly, you need confidence in your surgeon. If you are anxious about whether an operation will help or feel that the odds are not good enough, then consider getting a second opinion from another surgeon or explore other ways of managing your pain. Suggested questions:

1 What is the success rate of this operation?
2 What is the chance of my pain being completely cured?
3 What is the chance of my pain being reduced by half?
4 If my pain is cured or reduced, how long will this last for?
5 What is the chance of my pain being worse?
6 What other complications are there?
7 Will I be able to reduce any medications after the operation?
8 Is there any other way that my problem can be managed?

Remember, the answers to all these questions may not be available. This does not mean that you should not go ahead with surgery. Have realistic expectations and if a cure is unlikely, prepare yourself mentally and physically to manage any pain that remains after surgery.

Treatments for Chronic Pain

I f pain lasts for more than a few days most people will go to their doctor and seek help. The cause of the pain may be immediately clear to the doctor. Often, however, tests and investigations are needed. At this stage the pain is best thought of as acute pain and usually settles without treatment. People may take medication or use simple methods such as heat, ice or massage during the period of recovery. These approaches rely on the fact that the pain was likely to settle anyway.

If the tests don't show any problems, your doctor will reassure you that there isn't a more serious injury present. It also gives the doctor a chance to consider other medical conditions that may be present. If your doctor has a clear idea or diagnosis of what is causing the pain there may be a suitable treatment that will settle the pain.

On the other hand, if the cause of the pain is not easy to diagnose, it is usually not easy to treat. In this case the doctor may suggest trying a particular treatment to see if it will help. If the doctor tells you nothing has been found to explain your pain, this usually also means that there is no evidence of active disease present, such as cancer. If your pain continues your doctor will advise you whether regular checks are needed and how often. The results of the treatment prescribed will also need to be assessed.

At this point there is an important decision to be made. Continuing to seek a cure for your pain risks feeling as though you are on a merry-go-round and being demoralised by repeated treatment failures. The alternative is to look at how to manage the pain most effectively. The ADAPT approach can help you to manage pain, possibly in conjunction with other appropriate treatments. Many people find ways to get on with their lives despite the pain, and without requiring expert help. Others struggle with the idea of managing their pain and continue to seek help or wait until someone comes up with a better treatment.

You might wonder why people wait for someone to fix their pain and reject suggestions that using the ADAPT strategies could help. Often the reason they give is that they are not prepared to live with their pain and are determined to find someone to fix it. Hope is important but by the time the pain has lasted more than a year or so, further treatments are unlikely to cure it. The pain may settle by itself, but we can't accurately predict when. In short, you will have to face learning to live with it for the foreseeable future. Which means you have some difficult decisions to make.

Understandably, it is often hard to accept that there may be no solution to your pain. But it may help you to come to terms with it if the common treatments tried for chronic pain are explained. In the following pages these treatments are described and brief discussion is given of when and where they can be useful, as well as their shortcomings.

Medications and chronic pain

'If pain persists see your doctor' will be a phrase recognised by everyone. Most of the analgesics or pain killers work better with acute pain as they can target the chemical transmitters that are released with tissue damage. Chronic pain is much more complex. Since there is usually no evidence of continuing tissue damage, different types of pain killers need to be considered. While these medications may provide some benefit they are rarely the whole answer. They will not cure chronic pain like an antibiotic will cure an infection. Long-term use of pain killers may lead to unwanted side effects. What's more, even if they do help, you may overdo activities and stir up your pain anyway.

To help make sensible decisions about tablets for pain problems, this chapter will describe most of the types of medication that people use for chronic pain. Some of the problems of long-term use of medications will also be discussed. It is recommended that medication which is not helping or is 'just taking the edge off the pain' should be gradually reduced.

Medication reduction should only be started after discussion with your family doctor or specialist, however, and this process should then be supervised by them.

Advantages of medications

1 Medication can be very effective in reducing pain, particularly acute pain.
2 Medicines are generally safe provided that they are used as directed. All drugs have side effects even if you stick to the recommended dosage, but serious problems are rare with most medications. Always ask your doctor about side effects and find time to read the drug information provided in the box.
3 Stopping a medication will allow the body to clear it from your system, so its effects are usually reversible.

Disadvantages of medications

1 **There are no drugs shown to cure chronic pain.** A chest infection is usually cured by antibiotics after a standard course. None of the drugs available has been shown to cure persisting pain. If a medication reduces persisting pain then it is usually recommended that it should be taken continuously.
2 **All medicines have side effects.** Mostly, side effects are mild, such as nausea, light-headedness and constipation. For example, a laxative is usually required with drugs like morphine and codeine as they tend to cause constipation. Severe side effects are uncommon but if they occur, admission to hospital may be necessary.

3 **New drugs take a long time to develop.** The process required to produce a new medication takes a long time. It can take at least 10 years, be very costly and the drugs are usually licensed only for particular conditions. This usually means that a new drug is expensive and may not be covered by the NHS.

4 **Drugs may interfere with your thinking.** Many people on medication report that they either cannot think clearly or that they have difficulty remembering things. This can occur with many drugs, especially morphine-like drugs, sedatives and anticonvulsants.

5 **An 'old' drug may be repackaged and sold under a 'new' name.** Morphine is available as two preparations—MST Continus and Morcap-SR—which are designed to release morphine slowly into the body. Both preparations are similar, so that if one makes no difference to your pain without side effects, the other is unlikely to benefit you. Thus, if you are offered a new drug by your doctor then it is wise to seek information on whether this really is a new drug and, if so, what the success has been and how common are the side effects.

6 **No drug is 100 per cent successful in everyone.** Although it may surprise you, a drug that works for one person in three is thought by doctors to be a good treatment. Unfortunately, you may be one of the two out of three for whom it doesn't work. In reality, many drugs are not as effective as this.

7 **Stopping medications can cause a withdrawal syndrome.** If you have been taking drugs for a long time, particularly opiates and tranquillisers, it can be very difficult to stop them as they cause various withdrawal effects such as sleep disturbance, abdominal pain, sweating and feelings of anxiety. These complaints are likely to be some of the ones for which the drugs were commenced in the first place. Drugs should not be stopped suddenly unless under medical supervision, since doing so may cause a severe withdrawal commonly known as 'going cold turkey'.

8 **If the pain is bad it may be tempting to take more than the recommended dose of your tablets.** Studies have shown that people often take more than the recommended dose of a drug even if the drug is not helping or only 'takes the edge off the pain'. Taking above the recommended dose is dangerous as it may cause major side effects.

9 **Dependency effects.** Taking medication can become an habitual way to manage pain instead of learning more helpful ways of coping with pain and the problems that it causes. If you feel you have no other options it is easy to slip into the habit of taking pills every day even if they don't help very much. As part of changing your approach to managing pain it is recommended that under your doctor's supervision you gradually reduce medications that are either not helping very much or are not helping at all. Learning and improving your skills at using the more helpful strategies covered in this book will help to reduce your reliance on tablets.

10 **Supporting activity which is not sustainable.** Relying too much on medication can result in overdoing activities and further aggravating your pain. This is unlikely to be sustainable. It is very easy to overdo things and break through the relief that medication is giving you. This can result in increased pain and more suffering. Once you are using the ADAPT strategies analgesic medication may be a useful aid but it should not be the mainstay of your treatment.

Commonly used medications

There are a large number of different drugs used to manage pain. The list of drugs described here is not intended to be a complete account of all drugs available, but rather a summary of those commonly used for chronic pain. Further information can be obtained from your doctor or pharmacist, and useful reference books can be found at libraries and bookshops.

Suggestions for Using Analgesics with Chronic Pain

1 Take the tablets regularly, at preset times and not simply when the pain gets bad. The pills will be more effective this way and dependency problems will be reduced.

2 Keep a diary of whether the medication is really helping. Record not only your level of comfort, but your level of activity too. Unless you are happy with both, then the medication is not enough by itself.

3 If you decide you would like to stop taking medication for your pain, discuss it with your doctor and draw up a plan with him or her. Cut down gradually, under supervision from your doctor. This reduces the chances of withdrawal effects.

4 Keep a record of your progress and reward yourself when you achieve your goals. You will probably find that your pain is no worse and that you will feel much better in yourself.

Analgesics (pain killers)

There are two main types of analgesic drug: those not like morphine (nonopioids), and those like morphine (opioids), which are often called strong pain killers. Non-opioid drugs (mild pain killers and anti-inflammatory drugs) act to reduce the effect of the pain-producing chemicals released after an injury. They are most effective for mild pain and tend to work quite quickly. Simple analgesics include:

- Paracetamol (eg Panadol)
- Aspirin
- Ibuprofen (eg Brufen)
- Indometacin (eg Indometacin)
- Naproxen (eg Naprosyn)
- Sodium diclofenac (eg Voltarol)
- Ketoprofen (eg Orudis).

All simple analgesics can cause irritation of the stomach and for this reason caution is advised in their use over the long term. While this is generally less of a problem with paracetamol, using more than the recommended dose (eight tablets per day) of paracetamol can lead to liver damage. It should be noted that even with the recommended dose there has been a report of liver failure if this dose is taken for some years.

With the opiates (morphine-like drugs), it has been known for many years that very small doses of morphine were effective in relieving pain. Morphine was suspected of mimicking the action of a morphine-like substance in the body. In the 1960s substances called endorphins and enkephalins were shown to be produced in the body and to act in the brain and spinal cord in a similar way to morphine. Recent research has shown that morphine can also act near the site of injury and relieve pain. Unfortunately, morphine-like drugs also have unwanted side-effects such as nausea, drowsiness, constipation, mood change and difficulty in concentrating. A new combined medication has been released that includes a drug (naloxone) to reduce constipation that may occur with oxy-Contin. After the first few months, the body may become used to the drug. This is called tolerance and the dosage may need to be increased. The milder opiates are often mixed with simple analgesics.

Common examples of mixtures of opiates and anti-inflammatory drugs or paracetamol include:

- Dextropropoxyphene and Paracetamol (eg Digesic; Capadex).
- Codeine and Paracetamol (eg Solpadol).
- Codeine and Aspirin (eg Co-codaprin). These can cause stomach problems
- Codeine, Paracetamol and Doxylamine (eg Syndol). Doxylamine is a calmative and, as a result, many people use this medication to help them relax and sleep.

Common examples of opiates (which vary in strength) include:

- Codeine Phosphate (usually known as codeine)
- Buprenorphine (Butrans Temgesic)

- Oxycodone (eg OxyNorm, OxyContin)
- Morphine Hydrochloride (eg Oramorph)
- Morphine-long acting (MST Continus and Morcap-SR)
- Pethidine
- Methadone (Physeptone)
- Tramadol (Tramal)
- Fentanyl (Durogesic)
- Hydromorphone (Palladone)
- Dihydrocodeine (DF-118).
- OxyContin and Naloxone (Targin)

These drugs are usually taken by mouth, apart from Fentanyl which is absorbed through the skin and Buprenorphine which is available as a tablet and a patch applied to the skin. Pethidine is normally given by injection. In certain instances, morphine can be delivered by a needle or by a tube connected to a pump into the epidural or intrathecal space near the spinal cord.

Antidepressants

There are two main types of medication used to treat depression, a common accompaniment of chronic pain: tricyclic antidepressants and newer antidepressants. Tricyclic antidepressants are used to lift mood, help with sleep and may reduce pain. In most cases with people who have chronic pain, the typical doses (often 75 mg or less per day) of the tricyclic drugs used are well below the amounts (often more than 200 mg per day) used with people who are profoundly depressed. These drugs can be helpful for sleep and for pain at these lower doses and the higher doses are not necessary.

Common examples include:

- Amitriptyline (eg Lentizol)
- Clomipramine (eg Anafranil)
- Dothiepin (eg Prothiaden)
- Doxepin (eg Sinequan)
- Imipramine (eg Tofranil).

Some people with chronic pain find these tablets to be helpful. Side effects such as weight gain, constipation, blurred vision, dry mouth and drowsiness the following morning can be a problem. Concentration and judgment can also be affected and thinking may be clouded. Difficulty urinating may also occur. These drugs interact with tranquillisers, sleeping pills and alcohol, and can cause drowsiness. It is recommended that they are taken in the evening as they are likely to make people feel drowsy if taken during the daytime.

The newer antidepressants form a mixed group but most people know them by their trade names:

- Fluoxetine (Prozac, Oxactin)
- Sertraline (Lustral)
- Citalopram (Cipramil)
- Venlafaxine (Efexor)
- Nefazodone (Dutonin)
- Moclobemide (Manerix)
- Fluvoxamine (Faverin).
- Desvenlafaxine (Prisiq) / Duloxetine (Cymbalta)

These drugs have been shown to be effective in the treatment of depression and many doctors prefer them to the older, tricyclic antidepressants as they have different side effects. However, this also means they lack the tendency to promote sleep that may be seen as a helpful feature of the tricyclic antidepressants. So if you are taking the newer antidepressant drugs and you have sleep difficulties you will be advised to take them in the mornings. Some of these newer antidepressants have a benefit in reducing neuropathic pain particularly Duloxetine, which has been recommended as a first line treatment for diabetic neuropathy. You should be aware that all antidepressants carry an increased risk of suicide and suicidal thoughts so make sure you discuss this with your doctor and ensure that those close to you are aware and that they know what symptoms and signs to look out for.

It should always be remembered that drugs like the

antidepressants may not be enough to fully treat depression. Since they cannot teach you how to deal with stressful events in your life, including managing pain, you may well need to use the sorts of self-help methods outlined in this book. Many depressed people benefit from seeing a specialist in psychological therapies, such as a psychiatrist or clinical psychologist. A description of some of the most useful psychological therapies is provided on pages 72–75.

Sedatives
- Common examples of sedatives include:
- Diazepam (eg Valium)
- Nitrazepam (eg Mogadon)
- Temazepam (eg Normison)
- Lorazepam (eg Ativan)
- Clonazepam (eg Rivotril)

These are often prescribed as a short-term treatment to help improve sleep and to calm you down. But you may feel less alert and more tired during the daytime, and this can result in your feeling more depressed and reduce your sense of control. At night they may be effective in promoting sleep in the short term, but they can disturb the sleeping pattern over the longer period. As your body can become used to them, they are likely to become less effective. This is sometimes treated with an increase in dosage. If you are not careful the same thing will happen again and before long you can be taking a very high dosage without any real benefit. Trying to come off these drugs can then cause a withdrawal syndrome which can be an unpleasant and even a dangerous experience.

Some people report taking these drugs at the same dose for many years and swear they help their sleep or 'nerves'. However, in these cases it is most likely that their body is so used to them that there is no real chemical effect anymore. Any perceived benefit is likely to be due to the person's beliefs. However, withdrawal effects can still occur when someone such as this tries to stop taking them. If you would like to stop taking these drugs you should discuss it with your doctor.

These drugs also make it difficult to explore and challenge your feelings and thoughts. If this cannot be done then it is hard to progress to learning more helpful thoughts, which is an essential component of the ADAPT approach to pain management.

Anticonvulsants

Common examples of anticonvulsants include:

- Carbamazepine (eg Tegretol)
- Sodium Valproate (eg Epilim)
- Gabapentin (Neurontin).
- Pregabalin (Lyrica)

These drugs are called anticonvulsants because they were initially developed to manage epilepsy. It was then discovered that they had other beneficial effects, including reduction of some types of pain. These drugs are taken by mouth and are thought to act on the spinal cord and brain to block messages that occur with nerve injury or neuropathic pain. They also have a helpful effect on mood in some people but are also associated with an increased risk of suicide and suicidal thoughts. Unfortunately, they do not work in all types of pain nor in everyone with neuropathic pain.

Steroids

Steroids may be given in different ways but the usual way is by mouth. They are frequently used in chronic conditions such as rheumatoid arthritis to reduce inflammation. In chronic pain they are sometimes given into joints or into the epidural space. Long-term or frequent administration can cause problems, particularly with osteoporosis.

Local anaesthetics

Common examples of local anaesthetics are:
- Lignocaine (eg Xylocaine)
- Bupivacaine (eg Marcain).
- Ropivacaine (Naropin)

These drugs act on nerves and the spinal cord to block the transmission of the pain messages. They cannot be taken by mouth. Lignocaine may be given either by injection near a nerve, into a vein or under the skin. These drugs can relieve many types of pain but do leave a numb area and may cause weakness. They are usually not appropriate for long-term use (except in cancer).

Surgery

People have surgery for different reasons. One of the most common reasons is to try to reduce pain. In the past a general surgeon could perform most operations, but now they have become highly specialised. For example, there are now surgeons who operate only on shoulders and others who are expert in problems around the ankle. New research and ideas have grown out of this and today there are more and more options for dealing with pain in a certain part of the body. A note of caution. New operations are like new medications. You have to be careful of 'miracle cures' until a treatment has been fully assessed by eminent doctors and scientists in carefully controlled studies in more than one hospital or clinic.

Advantages of surgery

Surgery can cure pain but its success depends on having a clear idea of what is causing the pain. For certain conditions, such as appendicitis and a meniscal tear in the knee, surgery has an excellent success rate at curing pain and improving function. I recall as a junior doctor talking to a lady after her hip replacement. She had been in pain for many years and was particularly disturbed by it at night. The morning after surgery she was 'over the moon' because she had slept through the night without pain as a result of her new hip. Surgical success depends on having a clear idea of what is causing the pain.

Disadvantages of surgery

1 Surgery can make the pain worse. Many patients attending pain clinics report that their pain is worse after the operation. There

is a saying: 'there is no pain that cannot be made worse by an operation.' There is a strong element of truth in this. Some of the reasons for this are discussed in Chapter 3. If your pain is no better or worse after surgery then discuss this with your surgeon. Consider your options with the surgeon and your family doctor. This book should provide some helpful approaches.

2 Surgery is rarely 100 per cent successful. Minor operations can be very successful, but the 'bigger' and more difficult the operation the more chance there is of problems.

3 There are many common and rare complications that can occur during surgery and while you are recovering. Improved anaesthetic techniques and surgical skills are helping to make these less common, but they do still happen.

4 You may still need medications after surgery. Some pain may remain and you may feel that you still need to take medication.

Main types of surgery

It is not possible to cover all the operations that are performed for pain. Since back pain and back operations are the most common types of surgery, they are covered in some detail here.

Spinal surgery

Many patients with back pain are referred to a spinal surgeon— either an orthopaedic surgeon or a neurosurgeon. The role of surgery in this area is often controversial, however. For example, a number of studies have found marked variations in the frequency of back surgery between countries and even from one part of a state to another. Back surgery in the United States is far more common than it is in Australia or the United Kingdom, yet the same problems are seen in each country. Sometimes, patients with persistent back pain are so desperate for help that the surgeon may feel pressured to operate although there is no clear indication for surgery. There is no doubt that certain types of back pain can be helped by surgery but it is not certain who is going to do well. In general, back operations are only successful where there is a clear cut cause for the pain. This must be based on an assessment by a specialist doctor and complemented by tests such as a myelogram, CT scan or MRI scan.

There are two main types of spinal surgery: a laminectomy, the discectomy, and a fusion. During a laminectomy the surgeon removes the lamina (a part of the vertebra) to allow access to the prolapsed disc material. People often refer to a 'slipped disc'. This term gives the wrong impression of a hard disc moving and pressing on a nerve. What in fact happens is that the central jelly-like substance in the disc bursts through the strong fibrous layer that surrounds it. In turn, this may press on the spinal cord or nerves, causing numbness, weakness and pain in the area associated with that part of the spinal cord or nerve. Fortunately, most disc protrusions settle down without surgery, but if a bulging disc continues to press on a nerve, the bulging disc may need to be removed. If the surgeon is absolutely sure there is a bulging disc, and it has been shown on a scan to be pressing on the nerve, then this operation is usually successful (in 70 to 80 per cent of cases for buttock and leg pain). Success rates for back pain are much lower, however. A laminectomy is usually not successful when it is done for just a suspicion that there may be some pressure on the nerve.

A fusion is a major operation where two or more vertebrae are fixed together, either with bone or with metal rods and screws. This operation obviously stops much of the movement in the back, which after all, has a purpose. Fusion is successful in a small number of cases, but once again, it is not generally worthwhile when there is no clear cut cause for the pain or when more than two vertebrae would need to be fused.

As with laminectomies, the use of fusion operations for back pain is controversial. It is useful in some cases of cancer, congenital spine disorders and trauma to the spine, but it is less successful with so-called 'degenerative' conditions, from which most adults suffer as they age. Take this case:

Ruth had managed her back pain for years. So much so that at the age of 65 she had travelled around Europe on a bus. She had a lot of 'wear and tear' in her back and the spine had become bent. As she was getting older and she was concerned about the pain, she had a fusion where the spine was straightened up and fixed 'to look like new'. Unfortunately, after surgery she was unable to get out of bed because of her pain and the restriction in mobility that the surgery had caused.

In general, if a clear cause for back pain is found, the first back operation is the most likely to be successful, but second or third operations are usually much less successful and the pain could be worse. This means that if an individual has been unlucky enough to have an unsuccessful operation, further operations are unlikely to solve the problem. If a fusion is unsuccessful, however, a further operation may be recommended to take out the metal used for the fusion. This means another major operation. There are also many complications that can follow multiple back operations, including arachnoiditis where scarring occurs around the nerve roots. Unfortunately, very little can be done about arachnoiditis, which can be very painful. In some patients a spinal drug pump (see page 69) can ease the pain and should be considered but it is certainly not the answer for everyone. We have also found that even when these devices are helpful the patients function better if they use the types of strategies described in this book.

'Exploratory' operations

Before the high quality imaging available today, many people with persistent pain had what was commonly called an exploratory operation in an attempt to see what was going on in their backs. Remember, you cannot see pain when you do an operation, just as you cannot see anger or happiness by looking into someone's brain. For this reason it is often illogical to do exploratory operations for pain problems. If there is no defect shown on X-rays or other tests, there is little to be gained by an exploratory operation. Most of these operations are unsuccessful and are not to be recommended.

Surgery to cut nerves
A number of surgical procedures involving cutting nerves are used to try to relieve pain. They include operations on the spinal cord, such as cordotomy, spinal nerves (rhizotomy), and on smaller nerves outside the spine. It can be tempting to think that if pain is due to a compressed or damaged nerve, then cutting or destroying the nerve might stop the pain. Unfortunately, it is not as simple as that. For example, you would not expect to fix a faulty computer by cutting a few of its wires. Equally, it is unrealistic to expect to solve chronic pain by damaging the system further. In fact, most procedures where nerves are cut are not helpful for chronic pain. Operations where nerves are cut are usually recommended only for severe cancer pain in terminally ill patients, once all other options have been excluded. For example, cordotomy can be very effective for a small proportion of patients with certain types of cancer pain.

Radiofrequency lesions
This type of nerve surgery is one of the exceptions to the rule. The small nerves to the facet joints in the back can be interrupted by placing a needle beside the nerve which heats and selectively destroys it. Once the nerve is cut, the 'pain signals' cannot get through to the brain and pain relief may occur. Unfortunately, the nerve grows back. For this reason the patient may experience the return of their back pain after a period of three months to one year. While the procedure can be repeated, it is not known at present how many times this can be done safely. It should also be emphasised that this procedure has only been shown to be helpful in a small group of patients with spinal pain who meet stringent selection criteria after undergoing a series of nerve blocks in the spine.

It can also be successful in some types of facial pain (eg 'tic douloureux' or trigeminal neuralgia) where the application of this technique to the trigeminal nerve can ease the pain in the majority of cases for up to several years. However, it should be stressed that this treatment is only effective in a specific type of facial pain and it is not recommended for all persisting facial pain problems.

Injections

There are three types of injections used to treat chronic pain:

1 Local anaesthetic injection. These types of injections are also known as 'nerve blocks'. For someone with persistent pain, it can be useful to see the effect of injecting a local anaesthetic on a selected nerve. The effect can tell the doctor which nerves are involved in the pain. Sometimes local anaesthetic injections are also helpful in relieving persistent pain. In particular, blocks such as epidurals or facet joint injections can sometimes help back pain. Many people with chronic back pain get no benefit from these injections, however. In general, the longer the person has had the pain, the less successful the treatment will be. Although the risk of damage from the injection is very low, some people do report being worse off afterwards.

2 Steroid injections. Steroids are anti-inflammatory drugs which are often added to injections in an attempt to cure the problem. They are not a 'miracle cure', and they certainly don't work for everyone. While steroid injections may be helpful, they cannot be repeated very often.

3 Phenol injections. Phenol is a drug that damages nerve tissue. It is used to try to destroy the nerve in the hope that it will relieve the pain. There are two problems with this. First, phenol doesn't always totally destroy the nerve, so you can be left with a partially damaged nerve. If the pain is due to damaged nerves anyway, it is not surprising that this sometimes makes matters

worse. Second, as mentioned earlier, destroying a nerve may not relieve the pain. There are a few occasions when a phenol nerve block can be of value, however, especially when the pain is due to cancer.

Spinal drug pumps

Specialised pumps can be placed under the skin to deliver small quantities of a drug, usually morphine (and sometimes a non-morphine drug like Clonidine), into the fluid around the spinal cord. At least two hundred times more morphine would need to be given by mouth to try to achieve the same effect. This approach can avoid many of the side effects by limiting the dose of morphine. The drug is then carried to the spinal cord to block specific pain receptors, which can have a very powerful effect on pain in certain circumstances. Surprisingly, the reduction in pain is not always associated with increases in function and mood. It can be particularly useful for some types of cancer pain and in a small proportion of patients with pain due to nerve injury, including spinal cord injury. The main risks are infection, loss of menstruation in females and impotence in males. This technique is not suitable for everyone and is normally only done in carefully selected cases. Frequently, as with drugs taken by mouth, the patient with a morphine pump will still benefit greatly from using the types of strategies outlined in this book.

Physiotherapy

Passive physiotherapy

A number of techniques are used by physiotherapists for pain problems. Passive techniques involve the physiotherapist doing something to the patient. Examples of these techniques include manipulation, massage, diathermy, interferential, ultrasound, and hot and cold packs. While these techniques can be helpful for acute pain problems, they are not effective for chronic pain. Any help they may provide is usually short-lived. There is a possibility that you can become more disabled as you wait for the treatment to fix you. Passive treatments risk keeping your attention on the pain and its relief rather than working on things that you can do for yourself. In the long run, as you can't take your physiotherapist home with you, it is what you do that matters.

Active physiotherapy

Active physiotherapy is quite different from passive techniques. It involves trying to get the body moving again and also deals with building up strength and fitness. As you will already know, getting stiff and weak is a common problem with chronic pain. Active physiotherapy helps the patient to get the body going again, to get the joints moving, and to build up the muscles. If the patient is in poor physical condition, the exercises involved need to be built up slowly and thoroughly. While it may not cure the pain, active physiotherapy plays a vital part in helping chronic pain patients get back to normal life again. Active physiotherapy has also been shown to be helpful in preventing people with acute back pain from slipping into disabled lifestyles.

Stimulation

Acupuncture
The use of small needles inserted into the surface of the skin has long been used to obtain pain relief. In recent years the use of acupuncture in western countries has steadily increased. It can be a helpful treatment for many non-specific painful conditions, such as stiff shoulders and tennis elbow. Acupuncture does not cure chronic pain, however. Some patients do find that they get pain relief for short periods, but they have to keep going for treatment regularly. A typical course of treatment is weekly visits for six to ten weeks. Follow-up sessions, however, are often needed. Unfortunately, like so many treatments, acupuncture is not the total answer for chronic pain.

TENS (Transcutaneous Electrical Nerve Stimulation)

As you will recall from the discussion in Chapter 3 on the 'gate' mechanism in the spinal cord (see page 33), the 'gate' can be closed by stimulation of the nerves that carry touch sensations. Closing the gate mechanism in the spinal cord can relieve pain to some extent. This is why rubbing your knee or skin after you bump it can ease the pain. TENS works along the same lines.

Powered by battery, the TENS machine delivers small electrical impulses to the skin by electrodes that are attached to the skin. The electrical impulses stimulate the nerves and it is thought that this closes the gate in the spinal cord and so reduces the pain. TENS does not work with all pain problems but it is worth giving it a good try. You should be shown how to use it by a trained person. Most patients with chronic pain find that if it does help to begin with, it gets less effective as time goes on. Remember, it is not a cure. For best results with TENS you should combine it with the exercises and techniques in this book, in particular, pacing.

Dorsal Column Stimulation (spinal cord stimulation)

This is a type of TENS unit which can be implanted under the skin and is connected to a number of small electrical terminals near the spinal cord. It works along similar lines to TENS and is also powered by battery. This treatment is most useful when the pain is in one or both legs and is a result of nerve injury. It is less effective for back pain. More recently it has been used for pains in other parts of the body such as arm pain and the pain that occurs if not enough blood gets to the heart or the legs (ischaemic pain). Like TENS, however, it doesn't work for everyone. Even when it does reduce the pain to begin with, it may lose some of its effectiveness after three to four months. Patients who have had the unit put in may also suffer complications, such as wires breaking or infections. As a result, the units may have to be adjusted, replaced or even removed, which takes another operation to fix. Overall, dorsal column stimulators are not recommended for most pain syndromes but can be useful in carefully selected cases.

As with all treatments that can ease pain, you should not rely on these devices or drugs alone for the best results. The ADAPT methods described in this book should be the mainstay of your pain management plan. Drugs, devices or implants should be seen as aids to the things that you do yourself to manage the pain.

Peripheral Field Stimulation

In selected cases the electrodes used in Dorsal Column Stimulation can be inserted under the skin near the painful area and still be successful. This has been used for many painful conditions such as back pain, pain after hernia surgery and headaches. This avoids the risk of nerve injury when the electrodes are placed near the spinal cord.

Psychological treatments

Most of these treatments are provided as part of a 'pain management package'; that is, they can be combined with interventions like medication and exercises. Often your physiotherapist or doctor will use these methods as part of their treatment too, so it is not always necessary to see a psychologist for psychological treatments.

Hypnosis

Hypnosis is like relaxation except that it is usually performed by a therapist who speaks to you in ways that can help you to become calmer and more relaxed than you can achieve by yourself. You remain awake and aware of what is going on around you in the room, but noises such as the telephone ringing may not bother you as much as usual.

Once you are relaxed, the therapist or hypnotist will also make various suggestions that can help you to take your mind off the pain or even to change the way it feels. For example, under hypnosis the painful area can be made to feel numb or just a pleasant warm feeling, like you might feel after a day in the sun.

While hypnosis can be pleasant, it is not a cure. Like many other treatments, it only works for a short time (an hour or two at most) and so is not very useful for chronic pain. It also requires a therapist, which can make it expensive. You can be taught to hypnotise yourself, but that doesn't offer any advantages over simply learning how to relax yourself.

Relaxation

Relaxation is very similar to hypnosis (and meditation). You can use a relaxation exercise to calm yourself, to help you cope with pain, and to help you sleep. You can be taught to do it by a trained therapist or by using a tape recording. But in the end, whether or not you become good at relaxation depends on how much you practise it. Relaxation is really just a skill, like playing tennis or singing. Like all skills, practice makes perfect.

Relaxation is most helpful if you learn to do it anywhere. If you become reasonably good at it, you should be able to take the edge off the pain whenever it starts getting stirred up. In the long run, relaxation will help you more than tranquillisers. Of course, you won't stop the pain with relaxation, but relaxation can help you to cope better and to feel more in control.

Cognitive therapy

Cognitive therapy is aimed at helping you to work out ways of coping better with pain (and other problems, such as depression and stress by changing unhelpful responses). We all react to pain in different ways. Sometimes, the ways we react can become part of the problem and can make the pain harder to deal with it. For example, if you often find yourself getting upset and grumpy with the pain, you not only have pain to deal with but you also have to deal with being upset and grumpy.

It could be that your distress is more the result of the way you are thinking than simply the pain alone. Thoughts like 'This pain is terrible. How can I be expected to do everything in this much pain? I'll never be able to do anything. Nothing works' may be understandable but they are also self-defeating and risk promoting a sense of helplessness and, ultimately, depression. The good news, however, is that they can be changed.

If you are getting really upset about your pain it is likely you are thinking about it in unhelpful ways. If you could stop and reconsider these unhelpful reactions, you might work out more helpful ways to deal with the pain. As a result, you could minimise your distress and improve your quality of life.

Cognitive therapy can help you to sort out problems such as these. It involves examining the ways you think and how your thoughts affect your feelings. If your current ways of thinking are not really helpful, cognitive therapy can help you to work out other, alternative ways of looking at your problems. Becoming proficient at doing this on a daily basis does, of course, take time. But with practice, this more helpful way of dealing with a problem can become a habit.

Because we are all different, this type of therapy works best if you are prepared to look as honestly as possible at your reactions to pain. Doing so will help to make the therapy more useful to you. Typically, clinical psychologists are the best trained professionals to provide the cognitive therapy, but some psychiatrists and other health care providers also use this approach. Cognitive therapy forms a major part of this book and a fuller account can be found in Chapter 11.

Behavioural therapy

Behavioural therapy is concerned with helping you to change the ways you do things—your behaviour—which, in turn, can help your mood and alter the ways you think. Behavioural therapy can also help you to learn new skills and new ways of doing things. Many people say that all this requires is willpower, but it is not as simple as that. We are all full of good intentions that we fail to carry out. By using what we call a behavioural approach you can work out ways of making it easier for you to carry out those good intentions.

Without going into too much detail, behavioural therapy is basically:

- getting you to specify what you want to achieve (in terms of what activity you want to do),
- working out a realistic way of achieving your goal,

- working out what might get in the way of this and how to overcome it,
- putting your plan into action and rewarding or reinforcing your attempts each time you try.

Behavioural therapy doesn't tell you what goals to work for but it helps you to work out how to achieve your goals. Naturally, it is not as easy as it looks. Behavioural therapy techniques will help you to learn all the skills and exercises taught on the ADAPT program. In fact, without the behavioural therapy part of the program, you would probably have trouble achieving your goals. You would certainly have more trouble keeping up your exercises and other skills.

Psychiatry

Sometimes people with chronic pain are sent to see a psychiatrist because they are very depressed or because no physical cause for the pain has been found and no physical treatment is considered suitable. In the view of some doctors, when no physical cause for pain is found it means that the pain could be 'in the mind'. In other words, the person is thought to be imagining the pain or exaggerating it, or even saying they've got pain when the real problem is depression or some other emotional upset. However, not all doctors (including many psychiatrists) share these views. Nevertheless, many pain sufferers think that being referred on to see the psychiatrist is tantamount to being told that their pain is not real.

Being referred to a psychiatrist is sometimes a cause of concern and uncertainty for the pain sufferer and his or her family. Therefore, it is important to clarify what psychiatry has to offer someone with chronic pain, as well as its limitations.

First, it is important to realise that, like all types of doctors, different psychiatrists hold different views about chronic pain. In large part this depends on their experience and area of specialisation. Some psychiatrists will try to assess whether or not a pain sufferer has a particular mental illness. If the psychiatrist doesn't think the patient has a mental illness, he or she will probably say that they can find nothing really wrong and will then send the patient back to the referring doctor. Of course, if the psychiatrist does think the pain sufferer has a mental illness—which may or may not be related to the pain problem—then they will offer some form of treatment. On the other hand, other psychiatrists (especially ones with a lot of experience with pain sufferers) will try to assess the way the patient is being affected by the pain and will try to help them come to terms with it. This type of psychiatrist could offer to work with the patient using the types of methods outlined in this book. Their aim is to help the patient to cope better with their pain.

And second, there are some specific psychiatric treatments that have been given to pain sufferers. These include:

- ECT (electro convulsive therapy) involves passing an electric current through the brain. It can be useful in some depressive illnesses but it is not helpful in chronic pain. In the absence of major mental illness, patients should not have ECT for chronic pain.

- Psychiatrists often use drugs to treat depression and other mental illnesses. Many of these drugs may cause unpleasant side effects which patients with chronic pain find difficult to put up with. Although some chronic pain patients find low doses of these drugs to be helpful, high doses are seldom of benefit.

- Psychotherapy is any form of psychological therapy that involves talking things over with a trained therapist, who may be a psychiatrist, clinical psychologist, counsellor or social worker. It should not be confused with simply getting advice from someone. Rather, psychotherapy usually involves a therapist helping a patient to make sense of particular problems or even life-long difficulties. This can help the patient to work out possible ways of dealing with these problems. Psychotherapy can be helpful to someone with chronic pain, but it may not be enough. Therapies that emphasise not just understanding but also changing unhelpful behaviour and thought patterns are more helpful in the long run. Nevertheless, psychotherapy can be a useful addition to the more action-oriented approaches recommended in this book.

Alternative approaches
(or complementary medicine)

There are a number of different types of treatment for pain which are offered by practitioners who are usually not medical doctors. These approaches may be called 'alternative treatments' by some and 'complementary medicine' by others. They include osteopathy, chiropractic, homoeopathy, reflexology, faith healing and aromatherapy. While many pain sufferers report having tried these types of treatment, it has been difficult to work out how helpful they really are. For example, if they were helpful was it because the therapist listened, spent more time, and seemed to understand more than a standard consultation with a medical doctor allows? Are these treatments better for some problems and not others? Do they risk causing harm? How long do the effects last?

The trouble is that this sort of information is often not available for many alternative treatments. In part, the difficulty in testing these alternative treatments is due to the fact that they tend to be offered on a private practice basis and can't be easily studied, compared to treatments offered in a public hospital. Many medical doctors are also concerned that the people providing these types of treatment may overlook serious medical problems in pain patients because of their lack of medical training. Thus, they run the risk of not only mistreating the pain patient but actually making things worse.

All this is not to say that you shouldn't try these treatments. Rather, you should keep your wits about you and make sure that you understand what treatment is being offered, what it is expected to do, what are the risks, how likely is it to help and how long should it last. Of course, you should also take the same approach to any treatment offered by a medical doctor or other health care professional.

One problem can be the cost. If you have to keep going back week after week for these treatments they can become very expensive. So make sure you can afford the treatment before you start. Alternatively, budget for a certain number of treatments and then stop and think if it is really helping on a long-term basis. Keep in mind that because of your pain you may feel desperate and be willing to try almost anything. If you are in this state you are at risk of making unwise decisions, so don't rush in. Take your time over your decision and discuss it with someone you trust.

The best approach

Unfortunately, for most chronic pain conditions there is no magic cure. Of course, there are treatments available which provide temporary relief, and they may be worth trying. Even so, the short-term effects achieved by some treatments do not return the patient to the same condition they were in before the pain started. People with chronic pain have to come to terms with this. In this chapter we have looked at advantages and disadvantages of different kinds of treatment. This will help people with chronic pain to make up their own minds about what to do next. At the same time, however, we are trying to help each person learn how they can help themselves. In the end, it is how the person with the pain thinks and behaves that will determine how much the pain affects his or her life.

Using Pacing To Overcome The Effects Of Chronic Pain on Activities

Earlier, we described some of the ways in which chronic pain can affect your normal lifestyle. This section will have a closer look at some of these effects and how you can overcome them.

A key strategy is to use activity pacing.

Chronic pain usually leads to changes in people's activities and the way they do things. These changes will vary from person to person, but a typical list would include the following:

- give up working or work on restricted duties
- do less housework or home-maintenance work
- overdo things (push yourself), then have to rest
- do fewer enjoyable activities
- do fewer social activities
- avoid trying new activities
- rest or lie down more often during the day
- take pain killers (or tranquillisers or sleeping tablets as well)
- develop sleep problems
- drink or smoke more
- avoid people or certain activities
- have more conflict with family members and friends

As time goes on, these changes can start to become habits – you can feel as if you are in a rut. By then it can seem almost impossible to do anything about it.

These changes come about in many ways, but a common story from people with chronic pain is that they push themselves until they feel the pain tells them to stop. Then they rest, possibly take one or two painkillers, and wait for the pain to ease.

After a period of rest the pain may ease a little and then they will get up and try again – only to find the same thing happening again (more pain, stop, rest, try again). After repeating this pattern over and over, they may also start to get frustrated at not being able to do many of the things they used to do quite easily. Eventually, this can lead to feelings of despair and to wondering if they will ever get on top of the pain.

You may also start to feel as if the pain is running your life. In fact, many of our patients with chronic pain say that the sense of loss of control over daily life is one of the worst things about chronic pain.

The diagram below summarizes a common picture that many people with chronic pain report.

A Common Pain—Activity Interaction

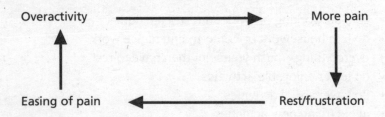

This pattern of 'overactivity-more pain-rest/frustration' can happen on both a daily basis and a weekly basis. For example, you may find you have "good days" and "bad days" (good days are when the pain is not so bad and bad days are when the pain is worse). What can happen in this case is that you will overdo things on the good days (perhaps trying to make up for lost time), but because of your lack of fitness you will strain your body, the pain will worsen and you will then spend the next day or two resting again (making yourself even more unfit).

Each episode of increased pain makes it more tempting to avoid doing activities which result in more pain. Over time, reduced activity (excessive rest) will cause the body to lose condition, with joints becoming stiffer and muscles becoming weaker. It might interest you to know that research by scientists working for the United States space programme has shown that even a week of rest can result in measurable loss of physical condition – even in healthy astronauts.

As your body loses condition it will gradually become less able to cope with a higher level of activity. Over time, less and less activity will be needed to overdo things. Rest or low activity periods tend to become longer, and total daily activity tends to get less and less – despite occasional bursts of high activity (which, of course, may end up causing more pain and then more rest).

The diagram below describes this common pattern of behaviour amongst people with chronic pain. It might be described as a life of "mountains and valleys".

Overactivity/underactivity cycle

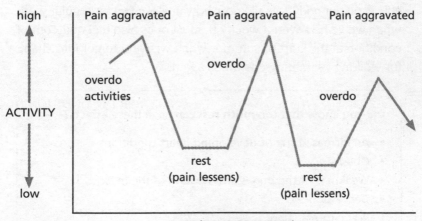

high

Pain aggravated   Pain aggravated   Pain aggravated

overdo
activities

overdo

overdo

ACTIVITY

rest
(pain lessens)

rest
(pain lessens)

low

TIME (DAYS OR WEEKS)

A classic example of this was provided by Ray who was determined to keep going with his old lifestyle, but this had still led to a "mountains and valleys" existance. On the 'good' days when Ray's pain was less, he got stuck into all the activities he couldn't manage when his pain was more severe. However, by doing more than he was used to his pain was stirred-up later in the day. The following day his pain would still be worse, so he would spend the day resting and doing very little, much to his annoyance and frustration. After a day or so like this, his pain would start to settle again and the pattern would be repeated. When asked what he thought about his approach, Ray said that he wasn't going to give in to the pain and he didn't want anyone to think he wasn't trying. But he also had to admit that his approach to beating the pain wasn't working and he was willing to see if there could be another way of dealing with it.

What sorts of effects can inactivity have on our bodies?
Naturally, this will depend on how long we are inactive and how little we do. Our bodies have a tendency to respond to the demands placed on it. Most of us have heard the saying "Use it or lose it!" This could apply to the risks involved in disuse of the body.

In a surprising short time too much rest can have quite marked effects on our body. We all know how unfit we feel for regular work when we've had even a week off. Most of us also feel quite out of condition at the start of summer when we want to get into shape for wearing swimming costumes again.

> **Did you know that too much rest can have these effects?**
>
> • An increased risk of developing heart conditions
> • Obesity
> • Weakness of the bones and wasting of the muscles
> • Depression
> • Premature ageing

Let's have a look at the effects of disuse on the main systems in our bodies.

Muscles and Tendons: A decrease in the thickness of the fibres occurs, and the tissue becomes more fibrous, causing it to become more painful when stretched. 8 gms of protein is lost per day with bed rest.

Joints: The cartilage in the joint, which normally acts as cushioning for the joint, becomes dried and breaks down. The capsule around the joint becomes tight and the joint loses stability due to weakness of the muscles around the joint.

Bone: With each week of bed rest, 1.54 gms of calcium is lost. After 6 months of complete bed rest, 40% of the body's calcium is lost. The bones rely on calcium for their strength. Loss of calcium causes the bones to become brittle and at increased risk of breaking.

Cardiovascular: This refers to the heart, blood vessels and lungs. The heart is a muscle, and if it is not exercised, it becomes smaller and works less efficiently. When you exercise, your muscle need more oxygen to cope with the increased muscle activity. The way the oxygen gets to the muscle is in the blood, via the blood vessels. The heart acts as a pump, firstly to pump the blood to the lungs to pick up some fresh oxygen and get rid of the waste products, such as carbon dioxide. The heart then continues pumping the blood around the body to wherever the oxygen is needed. Naturally, all parts of the body need oxygen to keep alive. At rest, the heart can pump enough oxygen filled blood around the body to satisfy the body's needs without too much effort. When you start exercising, you need to get more oxygen to the exercising parts. For this to happen, the heart has to work harder, the lungs have to expand more, and the blood vessels become more flexible.

Being inactive prevents all these cardiovascular mechanisms working properly.

As a result, • the heart muscle becomes smaller,
            • there are increased fatty deposits around the heart
              and vessels,
            • less volume of blood is pumped out of the heart,
            • the resistance in the blood vessels increases, caus-
              ing high blood pressure,
            • and the size of the red blood cells decreases. This
              means less oxygen can be carried around the body
              and you are likely to feel more tired.

Brain: • the circulation to the brain decreases causing
              reduced oxygen,
            • signs of tiredness and reduced alertness occur,
            • sleep becomes disturbed,
            • inability to cope with stressors increases,
            • and increased susceptibility to depression develops.

Genitourinary System: the kidneys become smaller because they do not need to filter as much waste product, and the bladder becomes smaller because it does not need to store as much urine.

Sensory: Bed rest has been noted to result in reduced sharpness of sight, hearing and taste. Balance mechanisms can also be affected.

All these effects have been demonstrated in people who have developed what some have called "**the disuse syndrome**".

Of course, no person with chronic pain will develop all these problems. But the list is a reminder of what can happen to all of us if we become too inactive. The list of effects should also remind you that not all your physical and emotional symptoms are due to whatever has caused your pain. They are not all a sign of underlying or undiagnosed injury. Rather, many may be result of the way in which pain has changed your normal lifestyle. The good news is that these effects are reversible – by your becoming more active again.

It is also true that not all people with chronic pain get into a pattern of overactivity and underactivity, but most will find they do less when the pain is worse and more when the pain is not so bad. If this is the case, you will still find that the pain disrupts your normal activities, even when the pain is not so bad. As time goes on the long-term effect on your body will still be a gradual loss of condition.

Why do people stay in this activity/pain cycle?
While most people will say they can see this pattern of activity is self-defeating, they find it hard to get out of it. After all, they can see how important it is to keep active and to lead as normal a life as possible – it's just that each time they try, the pain stops them.

Some people say they can't stop because they have no choice (eg. due to family or financial concerns). Others say things like: – "it feels better to finish the job" or "activity is often enjoyable, and it helps to distract me from the pain". Perhaps you will recognise some of these views from your own experience?

Other draw backs to the activity/pain/rest cycle
Besides leading to a gradual loss of physical condition, overdoing things then resting too much, then overdoing things again can lead to a number of other problems. These include:

- flare-ups in pain severity (which can last from hours to days)
- pain decides how much you do, not you (you don't feel in control of your daily life)
- it gets difficult to plan ahead because the pain might play-up
- working at a regular job is harder
- you can start to feel that you're never getting anywhere (and end up with feelings of frustration, failure, and even depression)
- having the pleasure of achieving something reduced by the pain.

How can you break the activity/pain/rest cycle and still keep active?

If you think you get into these patterns of doing too much/getting more pain/having to rest what can you do about it? Clearly, the first step is to realise that you do it. Then you should try to work out why you do it – perhaps some of the reasons mentioned above will be familiar to you?

Whatever the case, there are ways to increase your activity level, without stirring up the pain too much. So that you can once again enjoy a wide range of activities. Naturally, some activities will take longer to achieve than others. Realistically, you may have to accept that some are impossible. In these cases, you will need to look for alternative options or decide on your order of priorities. For example, if you can't do everything you'd like to do, then which activities can you drop for now? Remember, you may be able to get back to them at a later stage.

But if you stick at it, you can achieve a great deal. It is likely that even your doctors may not be able to accurately predict what you will achieve in the long run. For example, Jackie, one of the graduates of our programme had as one of her goals returning to work as an aerobics instructor. We felt this was unlikely and that she should set her sights a bit lower. However, she stuck at it and a little under a year later she wrote to us to say that she had achieved her goal. Her own words describe it best:

"I had been an ultra fit 21 year old jumping around, teaching aerobics, jogging 14 kms, weight and gymnastic training my days away, until one night I was injured while training. Having the mentality of a dancer, I pushed myself through am amazing amount of pain to keep going, so far in fact that I ended up bedridden for 2 whole years, experiencing constant pain down both legs to the ankles.

I was so desperate for a cure that I went everywhere, saw everybody, had 2 operations – both unsuccessful. The pain was enough to make me faint some days. I lost all muscle and went down to weighing just 36 Kg. Everyday was like living with the drip, drip of water torture. I was so depressed and in complete despair. I was in tears every day for 8 months. Things could not have been worse. I really believe no matter what lies ahead for me it will never compare to what I suffered.

After almost 2 years like that I attended the ADAPT program at RNSH Pain Management Centre. I was not confident that it would help and fought all the way about going. BOY WAS I WRONG !!! What a godsend the program has been. The commonsense approach to dealing with a chronic problem is now present in every moment of my day. It has become a way of life and the results speak for themselves. Not only has it helped me manage my spinal disc problem, but other setbacks along the way.

Now, just 12 months after the clinic, I am back living by myself, doing all my chores and would you believe, also working fulltime as a fitness instructor !!! I'm at university part-time too. Life has never been better.

The pain is still present to this day, but what I learnt through the program has taught me how to manage my life with the pain."

The key words for changing your lifestyle are:

– plan it – make it gradual – be consistent.

Pacing – an essential technique for mastering chronic pain

The aim of pacing is to maintain a fairly even level of activity over the day (as compared to doing as much as possible in the morning, say, and then resting for much of the afternoon).

There are three main aspects to pacing:

(1) Take frequent, short breaks.

Do something for a set time – then take a short break – then do a bit more – then take another short break – and so on. For example, if you can manage 15 minutes in the garden, but then have to lie down for the rest of the day, try working in the garden for say, 10 minutes, take a 15-30 minute break, then do another 10 minutes in the garden. This way you will do less than you could do each time, but you won't overdo things and ruin your whole day.

(2) Gradually increase the amount you do.
To begin with, it will seem as if you are going backwards, because you are doing less than before. But once you've got the idea of pacing, you can start to gradually do more. To "pace up" an activity you should plan to do a bit more each day or every second day. Each increase should be small and you should not do more than you planned, even if you feel like it. Before long, you will able to do more than before – and without the extra pain you used to get.

For example: To use the gardening example mentioned above, you would work out how much more you could do each day. You may decide to add on one minute more to each session. If so, on the first day you would do two 10-minute sessions. On the second day, two 11-minute sessions, and so on. In this step – by – step way you can slowly increase the time you spend in the garden, without overdoing things.

(3) Break-up tasks into smaller bits.
If the whole task is too much for you to try in one go, try breaking it up into amounts you can manage. For example, do three trips to the shops each week instead of one large buy. Or, divide your grocery shopping into two bags instead of one. As you get fitter and stronger you can gradually do more or carry more.

Guidelines for pacing
The three ways of pacing can be applied separately, but they will often overlap. Pacing should be applied to both exercises and daily activities, such as sitting, standing or walking. Whatever the task, however, you should follow the same basic steps to pacing.

(1) Work out what you can manage now

Once you have decided which activity or exercise you want to build up, work out what you can do comfortably now (without too much extra pain). This may take several attempts over a couple of days – until you are happy that your baseline is about right for you – even when the pain is bad. Try not to compare yourself with others (everyone is different). Most importantly, do not compare yourself with what you think you ought to be able to do (you are trying to work out what you can do now, not at some other time).

With some activities, such as exercises or standing, you can measure what you can manage by counting or timing. In this case, you should try the exercise or task two or three times and make the average your present level. You work out an average by adding the number of repetitions of an exercise and then dividing that total by the number of times you did the exercise. The result is your current average for that exercise. For example, if on the first try you can do 5 sit ups, on the second 7 and on the third 6, the total number of repetitions would be (5+7+6) = 18. You did the exercises on three occasions, so the average for the three occasions would be 18 divided by 3, which equals 6. Your current level for that exercise would therefore be 6 sit ups.

(2) Work out your starting point or baseline

To make success more likely, don't start pacing up from your current level (that may reflect a good patch). Instead, start just below it – at a level you know you can manage. A starting point 20% below your current level is a general "rule of thumb" we have used successfully. If you are not sure how to work out 20%, just reduce your current level by enough to be sure that you will succeed the first time you try the exercise or task.

For example, using the sit ups example mentioned above, you would set your starting point at 20% below your current level of six. This means you would start at 5 sit ups – which is what you did on your lowest attempt.

Using the gardening example mentioned earlier, you would set your starting point at 20% below the 15 minutes you normally spent in the garden at one time. This means you would start at 12 minutes.

(3) Decide on a realistic build up rate

Most people want to run before they can walk, but you will already know that trying to do too much too soon will make you overdo things. Before long you would be back to "square one".

You will be more successful if you try to build up your exercise or task slowly to begin with. Later, if you think you could go faster, you can give that a try. But first, build up slowly, then see how things are going.

You should try to build up your exercise or task at a steady rate, regardless of the pain. So, when you are working out your build up rate, ask yourself "will I be able to do that much when the pain is bad?" Of course, if you are too optimistic to begin with, and you set too high a build up rate, you can change it. But you will find it helps your confidence more if you set a rate you can keep up.

For example, using the gardening example used earlier, you might decide you could manage to spend an extra minute in the garden each day. If you started at 12 minutes on day one, on day two you would do 13 minutes, on day three 14 minutes, and so on.

(4) Write your plan down and record your progress

Trying to keep your pacing plan in your head will probably result in confusion and forgetfulness. You will find it helps to write your pacing plan down and to record your daily progress. In this way you will soon notice if you are making progress – or slipping back. Signs of progress will usually be gratifying and confidence building. You might even give yourself a special reward when you reach your goals each week. Signs that you are slipping or not progressing will give you a chance to work out why and what you can do about it.

Additional hints for using pacing

(1) Start on activities that are easier – Be prepared to leave those activities that are too hard for now. You can come back to them later as you get fitter and more capable. Start on activities that are easier. Once you have learnt how to manage them, you will find it easier to tackle the harder activities.

(2) For those activities that you cannot leave – It is most important that you still try to pace yourself as much as possible. Take short rest breaks as often as possible (stretch and relaxation exercises are helpful things to do when you have a rest break).

(3) Try to change your position regularly. For example, whilst preparing a meal, you could try to change between standing and sitting every few minutes, as well as take a short rest break every now and then.

(4) Remember, it is alright to **ask for help** with specific tasks now and then – everybody does it. People who feel unable to help you with your pain may be glad to be asked to do something they can do.

(5) Keep to your targets and plans as much as possible – This will mean that you (not your pain) decide how much you do. If you are having a bad day, try to keep going as you have planned but pace yourself more (ie. take more rest breaks). If you are having a good day, be careful not to do more than you have planned, to avoid overdoing things.

If you follow these guidelines you should have fewer flare-ups with your pain and you should gradually find yourself doing more and more. As the diagram below shows, this approach means doing more on the bad days but less on the good days (so that you avoid overdoing things). Naturally, this all takes quite a lot of discipline on your part. But it will be worth it in the end (which is why it helps to select goals which mean something to you).

Pacing up your activity level (step by step)

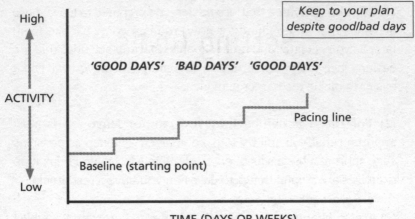

As you would expect, progress in this area is rarely "plain sailing". Set backs or flare-ups will happen from time to time no matter how careful you are. This won't mean you are back to square one, but how much trouble you have will depend on how you react. We recommend that you read the discussion on flare-ups (Chapter 17), but also discuss it with your doctor or clinical psychologist or physiotherapist.

How far should I go?

This is really up to you. In the end, it depends on what you are trying to achieve. For most people, simply achieving a reasonably balanced lifestyle, between exercise, leisure, work, and family or friends is enough. Others want to excel at something. But there is no point in simply getting fitter and fitter unless it is leading you somewhere. That is why working out your goals is critical.

Setting 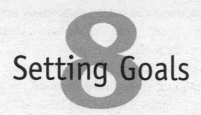Goals

Before you can start to manage your pain effectively, think about what you'd like to achieve.

What would you like to be doing that you're not doing now?

This chapter helps you work out these goals.

Goals are important because they provide the motivation for making changes in your lifestyle.

To overcome the effects of pain on your lifestyle it helps to think about what you want to achieve. Another way of putting this is deciding on your goals. If complete pain relief is not on offer, what would you like to achieve? What would you like to be doing that you are not doing now?

While many people may not think about their life in terms of goals, others do find it helpful to work towards specific goals. These goals may be things like saving up to buy a car or to put a deposit on a house. For others it will be to get a certain job or have a family. Goals give all of us motivation. After all, no one will work hard for a goal they don't really want. Goals also give us direction – they tell us where we are trying to go.

When you have chronic pain the obvious first goal is pain relief, then getting your life back on track. But if pain relief is not really possible at present, chasing it is likely to end up in frustration, wasted effort and, eventually, despair. Coming up with achievable goals can give you a sense of purpose and a feeling that you can control your life once more.

So, to avoid wasting your energy on impossible goals, it's worth putting some time and thought into working out a few realistic, achievable goals – things you should be able to do despite your pain. We call this process Goal Setting.

What are your goals?

Firstly, you need to work out what changes are important to you. Think of the things you have stopped doing, or don't do as much as you would like to. Often people have given up hobbies and interests, social activities, the "quality of life" activities, as well as work and daily chores. This can help you identify your long-term goals, or what you would like to achieve in the future. The best sorts of goals are:

1. Realistic

That is, they are within your financial means, appropriate for your age, skills, education, family situation, physical condition, and **can be done despite pain**.

2. Achievable

That is, they are things you can reach **through your own efforts**. They do not depend on luck or other people doing things for you. They may not be achievable right now, but should be over time, as your ability to manage your pain improves.

3. Relevant

That is, they are goals that **you** really want to achieve.

4. Specific or concrete

That is, you will know when you have achieved them. The most effective goals are those you can describe easily. For example, things like taking the family for a holiday at the beach or getting a job or walking to the local shops. Emotional goals, like being happy or relaxed do make life worthwhile, but are usually the result of other things happening (such as achieving your goal of taking the family to the beach or getting job). So it is difficult to make an emotional state your goal by itself. It will usually come from achieving something else. It can help if that 'something else' is specified.

Have a number of goals

It can also help if you have a number of goals to work on in different areas of your life. This not only gives you the chance of achieving more, but if one doesn't work out you still have others to work on.

Long-term and short-term goals

Long term goals are ones you expect to take a while to achieve. Short-term goals should be achieved sooner. Ideally, achieving a short-term goal should help you to achieve a long-term goal.

For example, if your long-term goal is to eat out at a restaurant, but you can't achieve that until you can sit long enough, then your short-term goal would be to gradually build up your sitting tolerance. This would continue until you could sit long enough to go to a restaurant.

As a guide to working out a balanced range of goals, fill out a LONG TERM GOAL sheet like the one set out here. This sheet divides goals into different types – Household chores, Family activities, Social activities and so on. Try to think of one or more activities you could use as long-term goals in each section. Remember the points made earlier – make your activity goals realistic, relevant, achievable and specific.

If you are not sure where to start, some examples of activity goals are provided in a list of possible activities at the back of this handbook. Your list doesn't have to be final – you can add to it as you think of other things you would like to be doing.

Long-term Goals

Household chores	
Family activities	
Social activities	
Recreation/sport	
Education	
Hobbies/interests	
Work	
Other	

Next Step

Once you have identified a few goals, you need to think about what is stopping you achieving them at the moment. Is it because you cannot sit or walk for long enough? Do you need to find out some information (important for goals like jobs, courses, etc.)? Or do you just need to get started and not overdo it? Try to work out the steps you will need to take to achieve your goals.

BASELINE (where to start) and **PACING** (step by step).

As was mentioned in the previous section on pacing, it often helps if you work out how much you are capable of doing at the moment – your baseline. It is often more realistic to work out how much you can do on two or three occasions, rather than just once. Then you can work out where you are now more accurately. Your baseline should be within the limits of your present pain tolerance – so don't push things to the maximum.

For example, if your long-term goal is to be able to drive your car for 3 or 4 hours, you would set your baseline by seeing how long you could drive comfortably now. Try to work out your baseline over 2 or 3 trips, not just on one good day. In this way you might find that on one trip you drove for an hour before the pain got too bad. On the next trip you may have only managed to drive for 10 minutes, and on the next trip it may have been 15 minutes. In this case it would be more realistic to set your baseline at something closer to 10 minutes than to an hour.

Once your baseline is established, you can set your first target, or short-term goal. **Short-term goals**, as mentioned earlier, are the stepping stones along the way to your long-term goals. You should not expect to get to your long-term goals in one day! The targets (or short-term goals) need to be stated in terms of how much you will do. To start with, we recommend that you start well within your capabilities. This makes it much more likely that you will achieve your early goals. Achieving your target will encourage you to try again. You can use the Short-Term Goals sheet provided as a guide to drawing up your own one. By checking off your achievements each day you can monitor your

Short-term Goals (Example sheet)

ACTIVITY	Mon	Tues	Weds	Thurs	Fri
1. Sitting	5 min	5 min	6 min	6 min	7 min
2. Standing	10 min	11 min	12 min	13 min	14 min
3. Lifting (floor to bench)	1 kg	1 kg	1.5 kg	1.5 kg	2 kg
4. Walking (in street)	15 min	16 min	17 min	18 min	19 min

Now draw up your own plan (make a number of copies as it will change with time):

Short-term Goals

ACTIVITY	Mon	Tues	Weds	Thurs	Fri	Sat	Sun
1.							
2.							
3.							
4.							
5.							

progress. Remember, this is often a good way to reinforce your efforts.

Using the driving example given above, you might set your starting point or first short-term goal just below 10 minutes – say, 8 minutes. Using the pacing method described earlier you would start driving for short distances but stopping regularly every 8 minutes. Each time you stop, get out of the car, do some stretching or walk around the car for a few minutes, then drive for another 8 minutes. Then stop again. And so on. You should continue this for 2 or 3 days, then increase the driving time and distance a little. To, say, 9 minutes, and repeat the process. After another two or three days you should increase the time and distance again. And so on, until you gradually work your way up to driving for 1–2 hours.

By increasing your driving time by a minute or two every few days it will obviously take some time to reach your goal, but you will succeed – if you keep at it.

Keeping it up

Your progress needs to be reviewed regularly. Your rate of pacing may need to be adjusted, depending on your progress. If you are having real difficulty reaching your targets, the rate of pacing may need to be reduced, or changed. For example, doing it a little at a time and more often may be easier. If you are achieving your targets easily, the rate of pacing can be increased so you reach your long-term goal more quickly.

Achieving your goals will be rewarding in itself. However, using small rewards along the way can help you to stick to your programme, irrespective of how you feel (whether it is a good day or a bad day). The harder a goal is to achieve, the more you probably need to reinforce yourself to keep up your progress. So, remember tell yourself how well you are doing (and doing it despite pain). Think of those tennis players, golfers and footballers you see on TV – when they make a good shot or a good kick you will often see them recognizing it by shouting or punching the air. You can do the same, but you may need to be quieter about it.

Finally, **stick with it!** Most goals can be achieved by working at them slowly and steadily (providing they were realistic in the first place). If you have continuing problems getting started or sticking to it, despite trying the above ideas, perhaps the goal is not really what you want. Or you're not ready to work on it just yet. That's OK, your goals are only there to help you achieve the changes you want to make when you are ready. You can always come back to them. In the meantime, why don't you concentrate on ones you can work on?

Recognising And Overcoming Obstacles To Change

I n this programme you will be trying to find ways of overcoming the problems caused by chronic pain. If persisting pain is interfering with your ability to achieve your goals or even to maintain your normal lifestyle then you need to find ways around it. Your goals may include such things as: giving-up pain killers and sleeping tablets, driving the car for more than a short distance, going back to work, doing more household chores, cooking a meal for friends or family, or just being able to play with your children or grandchildren.

As each person with chronic pain will face different problems, it is important that you should first work out the problems you want to deal with and the goals you want to achieve. [The chapters on Overcoming The Effects Of Chronic Pain On Activities and Setting Goals will deal with this in more detail].

Of course, achieving these goals will not be that easy (if it were, you would have achieved them already). You will face many obstacles. This section will deal with some of the problems you might face in trying to achieve your goals despite persisting pain.

1) Changing the way you've been living.

Some of these changes may be quite small, like doing some stretching exercises first thing in the morning. But other changes may be much larger, like attending an adult education class or even returning to work.

While you may be very keen to make these changes and achieve your goals, you may still find it quite difficult to break out of old ways or habits. Of course, if you're not quite sure if you do want to make these changes, it will be harder still. You may also say that "if only the pain would go away, then I'd get going". This is completely reasonable. But if your doctors have not been able to cure the cause of your pain, then waiting for it to happen before you get going could mean a long wait. The outcome is also uncertain – there is no guarantee that waiting 6-months or even a year would be enough. But that would be another year gone from your life. On the other hand, if you said something like "well, I won't give up hope of a cure, but in the meantime I'll see what I can do for myself" at least you'd avoid losing that time for nothing.

It would seem a good idea, then, for you to give some thought to why you want to make these changes and to how they might affect the way you've been living. What might you lose? What might you gain?

Another way of thinking about it might be to write down a list of the **advantages** and **disadvantages** of staying the way you have been and then a list the advantages and disadvantages of the changes that achieving your goals might bring.

Sorting out these issues may not be easy but it is very important that you do so and that you are as honest and realistic as possible with yourself. You may find it helpful to discuss this with your doctor or a clinical psychologist.

Your list of advantages and disadvantages of changing versus not changing could look something like this:

A. Keeping things as they are

Advantages	Disadvantages
At least it's the devil I know.	I don't like things the way they are, so I've got nothing to lose.
Change means uncertainty; I can avoid it by not changing anything.	If I don't give it a go I'll never know.
I avoid the risk of losing what I have got.	Things will never be any better if I don't try to change.

or B. Changing

Advantages	Disadvantages
I'm too young to retire, I'd like to do more.	There might be risks.
I could feel much better about myself.	What if I ended up worse off?
I could be much better off financially.	I might lose financially.
My family would be much happier if I could join in more	

Try making up your own lists then sit back and think about what they show you.

2) Fear of pain; fear of doing more damage.

Even when you're sure about the changes you want to make and why, you might worry that doing exercises or increasing your activity level could lead to more pain or even further injury to yourself.

How could you overcome these fears?

Information and reassurance? If you think information and reassurance would help, ask your doctor about your worries and read the sections of this book that might deal with your particular concerns (such as Chapter 3, What is Going on Inside Your Body When You Have Chronic Pain and Chapter 7, Overcoming the Effects of Chronic Pain on Activities). Sometimes you might find it helps just being able to talk through your fears and worries with someone else – even if they can't tell you anything you don't know already.

Do it – Once you feel reassured that you are not going to harm yourself, it can be very helpful to try and do the activity you are fearful of. Usually, it is best to start by doing a little at a time and then gradually do it more often. For example, if it was an exercise you were fearful of, you could start by doing it only once or twice (or whatever you felt you could do). Then, every second or third day or so you could do a little more of the exercise, until after a few weeks you could do it as often as you liked. By taking this gradual approach you will probably find that your confidence builds up as you progress (especially when you find that whatever you were fearful of didn't happen or wasn't as bad as you expected). Of course, as your confidence builds, your fears will be gradually overcome.

Use your relaxation technique – The relaxation and desensitising techniques you will learn during the programme can also help in overcoming fears, especially if you remember to practise them whenever you feel yourself starting to worry. [Read Chapters 11: Challenging Ways Of Thinking About Pain, 12: Using Relaxation, and 13: Attentional Techniques].

3) Time and motivation

You might find you don't seem to be getting anywhere when you make the first steps towards your new goals. For example, when you reduce your pain killers just a little you may not notice any real improvement in how you feel. Similarly, if your goal is to walk for 1 hour but you have to start with only 5 minutes you may find it quite frustrating to walk only a short distance before you reach your goal for the day and have to stop.

Even though your goals are important to you, they may take some time to achieve. You might think that it's just not worth all the time and effort, especially if the extra activities are causing you more pain.

How could you deal with these sorts of problems?

Your goals give you some incentive, but they may be too far away to have any effect to begin with. It may be like setting out to become a rocket scientist or accountant in a top firm – first you have to get into university. Then you have to complete a university degree or two in the right subjects. Then if your grades are good enough you might get a job in the area you want. On the other hand, it may take two or three job changes to get the one you want. No one ever gets to their ultimate goals in life in one jump. So we all need ways to keep going while we're getting there. How could you do this?

Will power? It's often not clear what is meant by this, but we may see it in famous sports people when they look very determined. Even so, how long do they have to keep it up? Usually, it's only for an hour or less. Perhaps a few days in some sports. In your case, however, you may have to keep working at your goals for months not days or hours. By itself, being determined is unlikely to last long enough to help you achieve your goals. Even top sport people know that. After all, they often have to train for months or years to get to the top. Will power may give you a start or help you at difficult times, but it's not going to be enough to keep you going. Other measures will also be needed.

List reasons for trying – One way could be to recall your list of the reasons why you are trying to achieve your goals (for example, how much you will enjoy being able to do more, how it will make things easier for you and your family, how much you don't like the side-effects of your tablets, etc.). You could remind yourself of these reasons each time you found your motivation dropping.

Break your goals down into achievable bits – If your ultimate goal is to walk for an hour, that might take a while to achieve. But you could break it down into, say 5-minute stages. So you could start with 5-minutes as the first goal. When you can manage that you would go for 10 minutes, then 15 and so on. In this way you could identify long-term goals and short-term goals. It's the same as the old idea of learning to walk before you run.

Record your progress – You can also keep a written record of your progress, like a diary or a graph. This can act as a reminder of your achievements and help you to see that while it may not feel like it, you are getting there gradually. The diagram below provides an example of this.

Sitting tolerance (how long I can sit still before getting up or changing position).

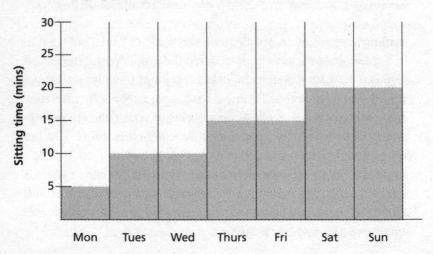

Give yourself a reward or reinforcer – You could also encourage yourself by giving yourself some sort of a reward each time you achieve your goals for the day. Such a reward need only be something small. For example, you could just give yourself a 'pat on the back' or a small treat – reminding yourself as you do it that you have earned it because of your own efforts. Of course, keeping a record of your progress may also be seen as a type of reward for your efforts – due to the sense of achievement you get from it.

Some people find it difficult to think of giving themselves a reward. If so, it may help to call it a **reinforcer** instead. This is a term psychologists use as its meaning is more neutral than 'reward'. In the rest of this book we will use the word 'reinforcer' instead of 'reward'.

Rather than use just one reinforcer all the time, we would recommend that you build up a list of several different ones – and vary their use. In this way you can avoid getting used to one and finding it boring. But remember, only use reinforcers that mean something to you. For example, one lady described how she liked to get up in the morning and sit at the kitchen table with a cup of tea and read the morning paper. But in order to reinforce her exercise routine she decided to only have her tea and read her newspaper once she had done her morning exercises. In this way she managed to keep up her exercise programme long after her initial will power would have worn off.

Even saying "I did it" or "well done, that's something I've achieved" is better then saying nothing or ignoring your achievements. It is even worse to criticise your achievements because they are not what you expected of yourself or what you used to be able to do – remember, you probably didn't have pain then.

Get your family or friends to help – You might also get your family and friends to help by reinforcing you with praise and encouragement whenever you achieve your goals (or better still, when they see you trying). In fact, it is more helpful if your family and friends praise you for what you have achieved, even if it's not perfect, rather than focus on what you haven't achieved.

In general, it may also help if your family and friends let you try to do some things first rather than do them for you – even though they might be able to do them quicker or better at present. Of course, you should discuss these issues with them first so they will understand and know how best they can help. Encouraging them to read this book is also likely to help them understand the programme.

4. Conflicting advice

If you have seen a number of doctors and other health care professionals about your pain, it is likely you will have had conflicting advice, leaving you feeling confused. Some may have told you to rest or "take it easy", while others may have advised you to "keep active". Some may have said "no tablets", while others may have said "take as many as you need". Some may have said you need surgery, while others may have said "don't even think about surgery". Whose advice do you follow?

There is no easy answer to this question. At times, they may all be right. But not usually at the same time. Deciding which advice to follow may be easier if you can understand why you have persisting pain. Reading the section in the book on medical aspects of persisting pain could help here. At least that will tell you about the sorts of reasons that can cause pain to persist and the treatment options with a reasonable amount of scientific evidence to support them.

It is also very important that you discuss the likely causes of your pain with your doctor. As mentioned earlier, even if he or she cannot cure your pain, your doctor should be able to reassure you that there is nothing seriously (life threatening or crippling) wrong with you. Your doctor can also arrange for any suitable tests or investigations to be carried out. Your doctor will also be able to discuss any treatment options with you. But if you are not happy with his or her advice, or find it conflicting with other advice, then you should consider getting a second opinion from another doctor. You can ask your doctor to suggest someone as he or she should not mind, and may even be pleased to have another opinion too. Your doctor could also refer you to a multidisciplinary pain clinic where specialists in pain management can provide a comprehensive assessment and advise you and your doctor on appropriate treatment options.

Your doctor should also be able to tell you about the possible outcomes of any treatment and any risks you may face with those treatments. An important rule in medicine is to do no harm. So, at least you could start with treatments that won't cause you any harm. Doctors call these "conservative treatments". Most physiotherapy treatments may be called "conservative". That doesn't mean they will help everyone with persisting pain, but they shouldn't make it worse.

At the end of the day, you will have to make a choice as to which advice you will follow. Whichever course you decide to take, you should try to be as informed as possible about the treatments offered, what they will do and what the possible drawbacks are. You should also check your progress yourself on a regular basis – are you any better or not? Is the treatment helping you to achieve your goals? If not, it may be that that treatment is not really helping you and you should see your doctor about stopping it.

You should approach the methods described in this book in the same way.

To conclude

By now you should have some ideas about why you would like to make some changes to the ways you manage your pain. If you're still not sure, then it could help to discuss it with your doctor or physiotherapist. If that is not enough, then you could ask to be referred to a suitable clinical psychologist or psychiatrist, or to a hospital pain clinic. A suitable clinical psychologist or psychiatrist is usually one who is familiar with the problems that people in

persisting pain have and the treatment options available. Even if
they can't offer you much help directly, they should be able to help
you talk over your concerns. This should help you to clarify what
you'd like to do next.

Stretching and Exercising 10

Health experts often tell us 'Don't take exercise seriously, just regularly'. This is all very well for those who are capable of exercising, you may be saying, but how could someone with ongoing pain like mine possibly be expected to exercise?

Many people who experience chronic pain tend to arrange their lives to avoid activity as much as possible in an attempt to lessen their pain. Is this sensible? At first sight it may seem so, because activity may be uncomfortable. A closer look, however, shows that taking less exercise is not the answer to the problem.

As you become less active you become less fit. This means that you can no longer exercise as much, and when you do exercise, it is more of a strain and often causes more pain. This can be the start of a vicious spiral of decreasing activity, as outlined in the diagram on page 112.

In the end the person with chronic pain may decide to give up many of their usual activities. They may give up their job, hobbies and sport. They may feel they can no longer walk with confidence, do the gardening, or even leave the house. As a result, they may become very isolated.

Exercises can be used to reverse this downward spiral. Of course, getting fitter doesn't guarantee success, but it can be a big help. Over time, getting fitter can help you to achieve an optimum level of physical and psychological functioning.

The Downward Spiral

PAIN

PAIN
(avoid activities)

LESS ACTIVITY

DECONDITIONING

PAIN ON MILD EFFORT

FURTHER INACTIVITY

FURTHER DECONDITIONING

PAIN ON MINIMAL EFFORT

The downward spiral

Athletes exercise to enhance their performance so they can go higher, faster and longer. Unlike machines which wear out with use, the body has a unique ability to repair itself. But to do this, joints and muscles need to be used, they need exercise. Otherwise they will become stiff and sore.

Fifty years ago people recovering from injuries, strokes, heart attacks or surgery were advised to rest as much as possible. Many were advised to stay in bed for weeks. But over time it was realised that rest was bad for these people. As a result, people with these conditions today are generally encouraged to get moving as soon as possible and to take up suitable exercises. Exercising promotes recovery, avoids the bad effects of rest and helps people regain near to normal function of their body.

In the early stages of recovery from these conditions people seem to accept pain in the short term for the long-term benefits which they know they expect to achieve. Similarly, it is a good idea for people whose pain does not go away to maintain at least some regular exercise. This can avoid the effects of disuse—muscle tightness, weakness, poor fitness and abnormal coordination.

The upward spiral

Being fitter and more active can also help you to feel good and improve your confidence in yourself. The diagram on page 100 shows how exercising can lead to being more active and feeling more confident.

You have already read in the Introduction about the difference between acute and chronic pain. It is a commonly held view that pain is always a sign of damage. This is true in the acute stage of a problem, when the pain is a warning sign that something is wrong. In the chronic stage, however, changes occur to the way pain is transmitted along the nervous system. These changes can amplify the pain signal from the original site of the problem, via the spinal cord, to the brain. In addition, the message coming down from the brain to the spinal cord is not dampening down the pain signal.

Once pain becomes chronic, it will fluctuate in severity, but that is normal and it doesn't necessarily mean further damage has occurred. It may simply be a sign of changes in the nervous system. Exercising is unlikely to take your chronic pain away, but it can help you to do more and to feel better than if you don't keep active.

The Upward Spiral

RETURN TO PRODUCTIVE
ACTIVITIES

IMPROVED CONFIDENCE

ENDURANCE ACTIVITIES

REDUCED FEAR OF ACTIVITIES

STARTING TO FEEL
STRONGER AND MORE
IN CONTROL

STRENGTHENING ACTIVITIES

START STRETCHING

PAIN ON MINIMAL EFFORT

Issues to address before starting an exercise program

Fear of pain

It is normal to be a little fearful of starting an exercise program. You may be concerned that if you exercise you could cause more damage, or you may just be fearful of the pain itself. By following the advice in this book, you will find that you are gaining skills and strategies to help you overcome these fears. Most importantly, as you increase your activity level despite your pain these fears will ease, especially when you see for yourself that nothing really bad happens.

Consider the case of Jane, who sprained her knee in a fall on some stairs and was fitted with a knee brace to support her knee. Because of her fear of the pain and the way she associated the pain with more damage, she avoided putting weight on her leg. This in turn meant that she started relying on a walking stick to walk and changed the way she walked. Eventually, the only way she could walk was to lean on the stick and swivel her body around to get the other foot forward. Before long she was suffering with back pain and a stiff and painful hip from holding her leg close to her body for protection.

At work she was put on light duties, which she found very boring. She was sleeping in a different bed from her husband because she was fearful of the pain if he touched her through the night and the risk of causing more damage. She had been having massage and heat applied to her knee and had been told not to move the knee if it caused her pain. The message to remain fearful of the pain had been inadvertently reinforced by the person treating her. No wonder she was fearful!

It should be mentioned that when anyone begins exercise after a period of not exercising, it is normal to feel muscle pain. This additional pain is to be expected and will settle as you maintain your exercise program and gain more flexibility and strength.

It is also possible that when you start exercising you may find that your chronic pain is aggravated. This is what you would often

have experienced after overdoing something. As will have happened in the past, this additional pain will also settle. Any flare-ups
in your pain through overdoing things will not mean that you have
caused yourself more injury. It could suggest that you have set your
exercise levels a little too high and you should start at a slightly
lower level. Have another look at Chapters 7 and 8 on pacing and
goal setting for more discussion of this issue. It would also be a
good idea at times like this to have a look at the chapters on dealing with flare-ups (Chapter 17) and challenging ways of thinking
about pain (Chapter 11).

One approach you could try would be to practice your relaxation
technique, do some gentle stretches, and decrease the number of
repetitions (say, by 50 per cent) and the level of difficulty of your
exercise program until the flare-up settles. But don't stop completely. After a day or two you could gradually increase your
exercises again to your pre-flare-up level.

As well as these steps, you should try to monitor the thoughts
going through your mind at this time—things like 'Oh no, something has gone wrong, some more damage has occurred'. If you
find you are thinking thoughts like this, you should use the thought
challenging described in Chapter 11 and try to turn your thoughts
around to something like 'I know my nervous system is oversen-
sitive and this is why I am feeling more pain now than would be
normal. I know it will settle. I've had it like this before. I should try
to keep myself calm. Use my relaxation techniques, check any
unhelpful thoughts'.

In Jane's case, she had several periods when her pain flared up
in the first couple of weeks of the exercise program. Over time, as
she applied the principles of pacing to her exercise program, she
could see that she could in fact do more overall if she timed herself to do shorter periods of activity, alternating with other activities
when she was not on her feet. However, she didn't wait for the
pain to become so severe that she had to sit down. Rather, she had
worked out her average tolerance for putting weight through her
leg, and had set a timer to go off at that time.

During these times when the pain flared up, Jane became quite anxious about what was happening. She found it very helpful at these times to write down what she was thinking, and then see if she could turn her thoughts to a more helpful way of dealing with the flare-up.

Acceptance

Another hurdle to overcome is accepting that your pain is chronic and that you have to learn to manage your pain. As we have emphasised earlier, before you can be expected to come to terms with having chronic pain, it is essential that you have been thoroughly investigated by the appropriate doctors for any medical or surgical options available to you. This should ensure as much as possible that there is no reasonable medical or surgical solution available.

Once the appropriate specialists have concluded that they have nothing further to offer, then it is a matter of accepting their advice. Of course you may choose to pursue the problem, seeking more opinions. But it is our experience that this can result in keeping you in the downward spiral of frustration and disappointment.

The case of Jane provides a good illustration of this situation. Jane's knee had been thoroughly investigated by knee specialists. There was certainly a minor problem showing in the knee, but nothing that any surgery or drugs or injections could help. This had been very distressing for Jane initially, because she wanted a cure. However, over time she came to accept that there was not going to be an easy, immediate cure. She also came to accept that she could benefit from seeking help in learning ways of coping with her pain and getting back into life again.

Goals

When you start exercising, keep in mind some realistic and achievable goals. Realistic goals for an exercise program are increased flexibility, strength, fitness and more endurance to do things without becoming so tired. Improving your physical coordination will help you to regain the skills necessary to perform many normal activities. Pain may be reduced, but it is more realistic to work towards functional goals rather than use pain relief as a goal. Functional goals are things that you do, like walking, driving, vacuuming and working. Seeking pain relief or cure from an exercise program would be unrealistic.

How can you plan to achieve these goals? If your goal is to pick up the grandchildren, you have to look at what picking them up requires. First, you will need enough flexibility in the joints of your legs to get down to the child's level. Then you will need enough strength in both your arms and legs to hold the child and raise your body weight, plus the child's, to a standing position. You will also need good trunk or back stability and strength.

An exercise program specifically designed for you would include all those component parts. Over time the exercise goals should be increased. At the same time it will be necessary to gradually include some lifting practice as part of your exercise program. This will help you overcome your concerns, especially if your original injury was caused by lifting, and will also help you to increase your confidence to perform the task, despite the pain.

Your lifting program would also be upgraded to work towards achieving your lifting goal of the weight of your grandchild. For example, this could be done by gradually lifting heavier and heavier weights.

In Jane's case, her goals were to stop using the walking stick and knee brace, return to her normal work duties and to have a family. Initially, Jane was examined by a physiotherapist and a detailed summary of her problems was prepared. She had some tight muscles, some other weak muscles, some stiff joints, some very bad postural problems and very poor balance and coordination. The advice about her exercise program was directed towards correcting the problems noted. At the same time, she started very gently to increase the time she could tolerate putting the weight through her bad leg.

At the same time, Jane started to go up and down stairs.

Remember, her original injury was from a fall she had going down stairs. Naturally, she was apprehensive about doing this activity, at least to begin with. As she got going these fears diminished and her confidence grew.

Remember, confidence grows out of doing things. Waiting until you are confident *before* you do things may take a long time and you may still not get anywhere.

The Purposes of an Exercise Program

- To reverse the effects of inactivity on your body
- To help you to do more of your normal activities
- To reduce your physical limitations
- To help you feel better and more confident about yourself

Remember, expecting exercises to get rid of chronic pain is generally unrealistic. The usefulness of exercises should not be measured in terms of pain relief.

Getting under way

Planning your exercise program

Like most people, you can work out your own exercise program or simply go to a local gymnasium for advice and equipment. However, if you are not confident about doing this or you have been inactive for an extended time then discuss your plans and goals with your doctor. He or she may advise you to have a general physical check-up, especially for your heart, first.

You might also find it helpful to see a physiotherapist for guidance. This use of a physiotherapist should not be confused with having 'hands on' treatments such as manipulation or massage, which are not generally useful in the management of chronic pain. Rather, the physiotherapist would be expected to give you a good physical examination to identify exactly which areas of your body are tight, which areas are weak, and what postural problems you may have. These imbalances may have resulted from your pain and subsequent inactivity and could be corrected by appropriate exercise and advice.

You will find a number of stretches and exercises described in the following pages, but there are many stretches and exercises for each muscle group.

This chapter will cover the main aspects of a typical exercise program for someone in chronic pain, but you might find it helpful to obtain specific advice about your problem from an expert like a physiotherapist. If you do seek advice we recommend that you take this book along to show the physiotherapist the sort of thing you are seeking. You should only need to see the physiotherapist two or three times to work out a suitable exercise program and to get it started.

Once you are confident about performing your exercise program, going to a gymnasium regularly can be a good way to maintain your program—if you like that sort of place (many don't feel comfortable in them). If you like swimming, or cycling, or just walking, then these also can be appropriate ways to upgrade your fitness. But you shouldn't work on these sorts of activities until you have achieved adequate flexibility and strength through your exercise program.

A stationary bike or treadmill can be a good way to start. For your swimming program, you would need to develop adequate shoulder mobility and strength and leg strength to be able to perform the stroke correctly.

Remember, it doesn't really matter where you exercise as long as you are exercising regularly.

Typical components of an exercise program
People who exercise regularly, from elite athletes down, use a basic format. They stretch, they do strengthening exercises, they improve their aerobic fitness which increases their endurance to avoid becoming fatigued, and they improve their skills to perform specific tasks by working on their coordination.

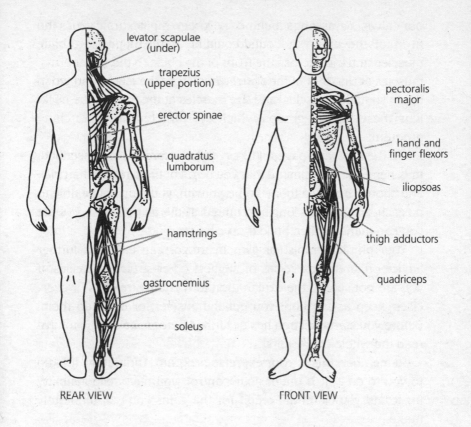

levator scapulae (under)

trapezius (upper portion)

erector spinae

quadratus lumborum

hamstrings

gastrocnemius

soleus

pectoralis major

hand and finger flexors

iliopsoas

thigh adductors

quadriceps

REAR VIEW

FRONT VIEW

Stretching

Stretching has the effect of loosening tight structures. When a muscle is gently stretched the fibres that make up the muscle elongate and relax. This allows the joints to move further. The structures in our body most responsive to stretching are muscles, tendons, ligaments, joint capsules, the sheath around the nerves, skin and fascia. Because all these tissues are somehow involved with muscles, it is easiest to talk about stretching 'muscles'.

The diagram above shows the muscles with mainly postural functions which tend to tighten then shorten. In our bodies, some muscle groups have a tendency to tighten. These include our calves, hamstrings (behind the knee), hip flexors (across the front of the hips), the outside band of the upper leg, back muscles, muscles across the front of the chest to the upper arms, muscles at the front of the upper arm across the elbow and wrist, upper shoulder muscles, and the muscles at the front of the neck. It is these muscle groups which are targeted in a stretching program.

On the following pages, 11 key stretch exercises are described. In general, we recommend that you do all of them rather than pick and choose between them. To begin with, you may not be able to do each stretch for as long as required. That's all right; just do what you can manage, then build it up over time.

Your physiotherapist or gym instructor can give you further advice on stretch exercises or suggest other stretch exercises. If you are not sure of the explanation for certain stretches or exercises, keep asking until you get the answer, or don't do them. Before you start the stretches described here make sure you have read the whole chapter first.

Remember, this is your exercise program. Ultimately, it is up to you to do it. It is under your control, you have responsibility for it and you claim the credit for the gains you will ultimately make.

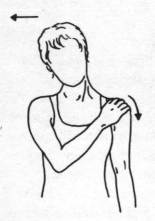

Shoulder-neck stretch
Place the right hand on top of the left shoulder and tilt the head towards the right shoulder. Shrug the left shoulder upwards for 5 seconds, whilst pushing down on the shoulder with the right hand. Relax the muscle, then push the shoulder down for a further 10 seconds, maintaining the head position. Repeat for opposite side.

Posterior shoulder stretch

Bend elbow to 90 degrees and use oppo-site hand to bring it across chest. Hold elbow against chest, but rotate hand away from body while maintaining the elbow position (that is, 90 degrees). Hold the position for a minimum of 15 sec-onds, and repeat. The best results will be achieved if this stretch is done three or more times across the day.

NOTE: *If at any time you are uncertain about your exercises, discuss it with your physiotherapist or doctor.*

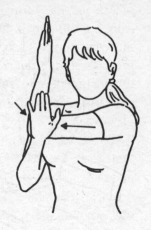

Triceps stretch

Raise your right arm and place your right hand behind your neck. Reaching over your head with the left hand, pull the right elbow back towards the centre of your back. If you have difficulty reach-ing over your head with the left hand, bring your left arm in front of your body and push the elbow backwards. Hold the position for a minimum of 15 seconds, and repeat. Then repeat with the other arm. The best results will be achieved if this stretch is done three or more times across the day.

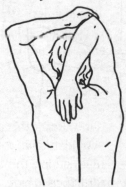

NOTE: *If at any time you are uncertain about your exercises, discuss it with your physiotherapist or doctor.*

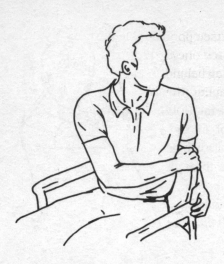

Spinal rotation

Sitting in chair, place one hand on the chair behind the opposite shoulder. Twist your body to look over that shoulder using the hand on the chair to pull your body around. Hold for 5 seconds. Repeat to other side.

NOTE: *If at any time you are uncertain about your exercises, discuss it with your physiotherapist or doctor.*

Pectoral and anterior chest wall stretch

Place hand against wall, fingers pointing backwards, thumb upwards, palm flat on wall. Straighten elbow and turn body away from wall gradually, until a pull is felt. Maintain for 10 seconds. Repeat for opposite side.

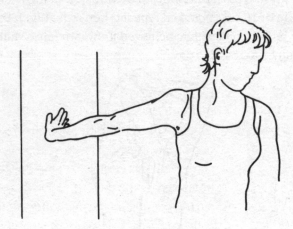

VARIATIONS: *Follow the instructions above, with fingers pointing upwards and thumb forwards; or fingers pointing forwards and thumb down.*

Calf stretch

Lean forward on to a stable surface (for example, back of a chair or the wall). Place one foot forward and straighten the other leg behind. Feet should be facing forwards. Keeping the heel of the back foot on the ground and the knee on the front leg bent, lean forward onto the front knee. Hold the position for a minimum of 15 seconds, and repeat. The best results will be achieved if this stretch is done three or more times across the day.

NOTE: *If at any time you are uncertain about your exercises, discuss it with your physiotherapist or doctor.*

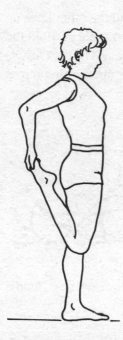

Quadriceps stretch

Stand on one leg, bend the other knee and grasp the foot with the opposite hand. You may need to use something stable for balance. Keeping the knees together, pull your foot towards your buttocks. It is important that you do not bend forward at the hips. Hold the position for a minimum of 15 seconds, and repeat. The best results will be achieved if this stretch is done three or more times across the day.

NOTE: *If at any time you are uncertain about your exercises, discuss it with your physiotherapist or doctor.*

Hamstrings stretch

Rest one heel on a support of a suitable height to allow you to keep the knee straight. Keep your back straight (that is, bend at the hips) as you lean forward towards your toes. Hold position for a minimum of 15 seconds, and repeat. The best result will be achieved if this stretch is done three or more times across the day.

NOTE: *If at any time you are uncertain about your exercises, discuss it with your physiotherapist or doctor.*

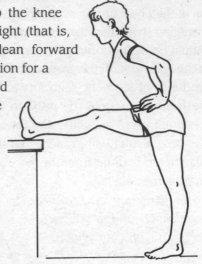

Hip extensor stretch

Lie on your back with one leg out straight. Bend the other knee up and use your hands to pull the leg towards your chest. Hold the position for a minimum of 15 seconds, and repeat. The best results will be achieved if this stretch is done three or more times across the day.

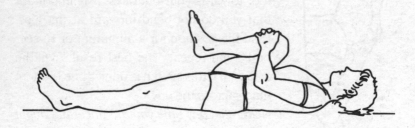

NOTE: *If at any time you are uncertain about your exercises, discuss it with your physiotherapist or doctor.*

Gluteals stretch

Lie on your back with both knees bent. Rest one ankle across the top of the opposite knee. Grasp the bent knee and pull it towards your chest, which at the same time will raise the other leg. Hold the position for a minimum of 15 seconds, and repeat. The best results will be achieved if this stretch is done three or more times across the day.

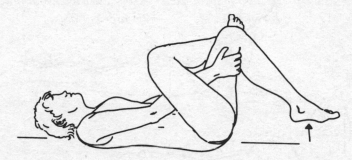

NOTE: *If at any time you are uncertain about your exercises, discuss it with your physiotherapist or doctor.*

Latissimus dorsi stretch

Start on your hands and knees, with your arms straight and your shoulders and hips at the same height. Gently rock your buttocks backwards until they rest on your heels. Slide your arms forwards until they are outstretched in front of you. Hold this position for a minimum of 15 seconds, and repeat. The best results will be achieved if this stretch is done three or more times across the day.

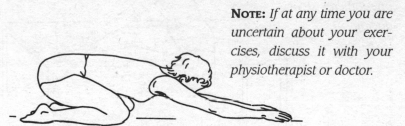

NOTE: *If at any time you are uncertain about your exercises, discuss it with your physiotherapist or doctor.*

Back arch press-up

Lie flat on your stomach on the mat, placing your hands under your shoulders. Without lifting your hips off the mat, push up with your arms. Your back and abdominal muscles should be relaxed throughout this exercise. Hold for 5 seconds then slowly lower your body, and repeat.

> **NOTE:** *If at any time you are uncertain about your exercises, discuss it with your physiotherapist or doctor.*

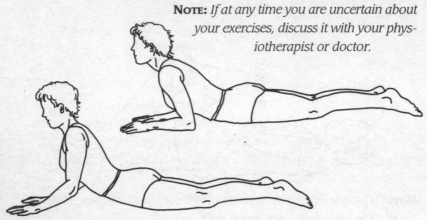

Sciatic nerve stretch

Sit with one leg along the bed or table, the other foot on the floor. Keep the knee along the bed or table straight, and stretch down with both hands to reach towards your foot. Pull your toes up towards you.

NOTE: *If at any time you are uncertain about your exercises, discuss it with your physiotherapist or doctor.*

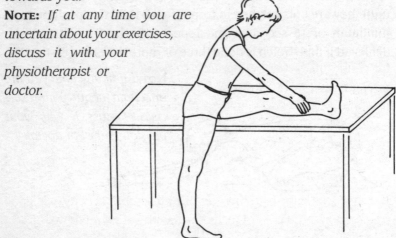

How long and how often?

You may have noticed that it is necessary to stretch regularly. If you have practised stretches for a few weeks or so and then had a period without stretching, you can feel quite stiff when you begin stretching again. This is because the tissues have a natural tendency to adapt to the positions in which they are used. Stretching beyond this point gives a sensation of tightness. Therefore, it is important to stretch regularly. This may mean 2–3 times per day, particularly if pain is limiting your natural ability to freely perform your full range of movements.

Holding each stretch for 15 seconds is a good time. Longer stretches may be more beneficial in some situations, but if you are suffering pain and you are trying to get your confidence to move your body a little more, then 15 seconds is okay. Of course, 15 seconds may be too much initially. In this case, stretch for as long as you can, but record how long you were able to stretch. The aim would be to gradually increase the time you are able to stretch.

After your first stretch, release the stretch, rest for a few seconds, then repeat the stretch. Follow this routine as you stretch all the muscle groups throughout the body. This should take about 20 minutes, once you are confident and familiar with your stretches. This 20-minute session should be repeated 2–3 times per day.

Warm-up stretches

Sometimes you may choose to use your stretches to warm up before doing your strengthening or aerobic exercise. Stretches are best performed when your muscles are warm. A warm shower can be a good way to warm up your muscles. Alternatively, you may like to warm up with a gentle walk before beginning your stretches.

Similarly, after exercising, it is helpful to stretch again to help relieve the after exercise muscle ache that sometimes occurs.

Stretching and relaxation

Because stretching is a slow, gentle and smooth activity, it is good to incorporate relaxation techniques with your stretching. As you are feeling the muscles let go in your stretch, you could try to breathe out slowly, just like you do in the relaxation exercise.

Strengthening exercises

Strengthening has the effect of making muscles stronger as muscle fibres get bigger. Muscle is the only tissue that responds to strengthening exercises. Strengthening muscles depends on gradually increasing the load on the muscle. This can be done by increasing the number of repetitions and/or sets of the exercise, increasing the length of time the exercise is held, or increasing the weight or resistance the muscle has to work against. Strengthening is different from stretching, which depends on the regular elongation of the tissues.

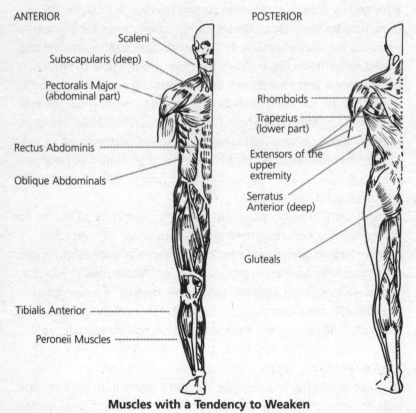

ANTERIOR

Scaleni
Subscapularis (deep)
Pectoralis Major (abdominal part)
Rectus Abdominis
Oblique Abdominals
Tibialis Anterior
Peroneii Muscles

POSTERIOR

Rhomboids
Trapezius (lower part)
Extensors of the upper extremity
Serratus Anterior (deep)
Gluteals

Muscles with a Tendency to Weaken

As was noted before, certain muscle groups have a tendency to shorten and tighten. Equally, some other muscles have a greater tendency to weaken, often simply in response to becoming inactive and not being used—not in response to the underlying pain problem alone. See the diagram above for the muscle groups with a tendency to weaken.

These muscle groups are the ones that help pull the body straight after the tight ones have pulled it into a hunched over, curled up position. They tend to be the muscles at the front of the shins, along the inside of the knee, the buttocks, the abdominals, the muscles between the shoulder blades, the muscles which pull the head back.

You may have noticed a pattern here. Muscles work in pairs across every joint. The aim of exercises is to have full flexibility and strength of both muscle groups across each joint. For example, when you bend your elbow, muscles at the front of the elbow shorten and tighten, while muscles at the back of the elbow have to lengthen. When you straighten the elbow, the reverse happens. Therefore, both muscle groups need both flexibility and strength. Imbalance between these muscle groups will cause a dysfunction to the quality of movement at the elbow, and may cause more damage at the joint.

The whole body works according to this principle. In the trunk and spine, the pair of muscles supporting the trunk is the back extensors and the abdominals.

Planning your strengthening routine
In order to plan the exercise program, it is important to work out which muscles or muscle groups you plan to strengthen. A professional assessment by a physiotherapist will help you to determine this.

An outline of a basic strengthening exercise program for the whole body is presented here to get you started. This program applies regardless of the site of your pain. Remember, the reason for these exercises is to help you do more rather than relieve your pain.

Strengthening Exercise Chart

Week Starting

	Abdominal Hollowing	Lower Abdominal A	Lunge	Step	Hip Extension	Hip Extension	Leg Lift	Chin Ins	Shoulder Retraction 2
BASELINE (Mon)	10	4	7	9	4	6	8	5	10
(Tues)	6	2	4	3	6	8	3	4	10
Start/Pacing	$16 \div 2 = 8$ $-20\% = -1.6$ $\overline{6.4}$	$6 \div 2 = 3$ $-20\% = -0.6$ $\overline{2.4}$	$11 \div 2 = 5.5$ $-20\% = -1.1$ $\overline{4.4}$	$12 \div 2 = 6$ $-20\% = -1.2$ $\overline{4.8}$	$10 \div 2 = 5$ $-20\% = -1$ $\overline{4}$	$14 \div 2 = 7$ $-20\% = -1.4$ $\overline{5.6}$	$11 \div 2 = 5.5$ $-20\% = -1.4$ $\overline{4.4}$	$9 \div 2 = 4.5$ $-20\% = -0.9$ $\overline{3.6}$	$20 \div 2 = 10$ $-20\% = -1$ $\overline{9}$
WED	6	2	4	5	4	5	4	3	9
THURS									
FRI									
SAT									
SUN									
MON									
TUES									

Name:

Before starting to upgrade your strengthening program, it is important to establish a baseline—that is, a safe and comfortable level at which to begin your program. See Chapter 7 for a discussion on learning to pace up your activities. Remember to break up large tasks into small bits, take frequent short breaks and to gradually increase the amount you do.

Use the Strengthening Exercise Chart provided on page 132 as an example. You can copy your own chart onto a piece of paper.

To set your exercise baseline, you should record the number or repetitions you perform of each exercise on the first and second day of your program. Remember to start at a level that you can manage comfortably, no matter how little. Don't push yourself.

Once you have two recordings for each exercise, you do the following calculations. Add the number of repetitions together. For example 6 + 4 = 10 and then work out the average of those two figures. In this case, 10 divided by 2 = 5.

Then work out 80 per cent of that figure (or take 20 per cent off the average figure). Eighty per cent of 5 is 4. This then becomes your starting point for your exercise program. This is your real baseline. The figure doesn't have to be exact, a rough estimate will do, as long as it is less than your average.

The reason for starting this way is to be quite sure that you are starting your exercise program at a level that is safe and achievable for you. From then on it is a matter of setting a gradually increasing goal each day or two (you have to decide which would suit you better). So you might increase by one or more repetitions each day or every second or third day—whatever you feel you can manage. Remember to pace.

The way you upgrade your exercise program depends on the effects you wish to achieve. Upgrading in different ways will achieve different results. If you want to increase strength and bulk in the muscles, then a method called the 'one rep max' is appropriate. This means that you lift the maximum weight that you can lift only once. A modification of this method may be to find the weight you can lift once, reduce it by 25 per cent and then lift that weight 4 or 5 times.

Probably the most useful method of upgrading for people who are trying to increase their activities despite their pain is to follow the principle of building up to doing three sets of 6–10 repetitions. The effect of exercising this way is to increase endurance and stamina to keep on doing things without becoming as tired.

Abdominal hollowing

Lie on your back with both legs bent and feet flat on mat/floor. Maintain the natural curve of your lower back. Breathe in . . . and out . . . then stop breathing for a moment and slowly and gently draw your lower abdomen in. Hold this contraction for a few seconds while breathing normally again. Then relax.

Do as many as you can and record the number on your strengthening exercise sheet.

The tendency will be to hold your breath, however it is important to maintain the hollowing while breathing normally.

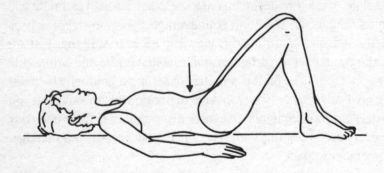

NOTE: *If at any time you are uncertain about your exercises, discuss it with your physiotherapist or doctor.*

Abdominal hollowing with double leg lift

Lie on your back with your knees bent and feet flat on floor/bed. While doing your abdominal hollowing, lift one leg off the ground, and then the other leg. Then lower one leg at a time back to the starting position. Then relax your abdomen.

The tendency will be to hold your breath, however, it is important to maintain the hollowing while breathing normally throughout this exercise.

NOTE: *If at any time you are uncertain about your exercises, discuss it with your physiotherapist or doctor.*

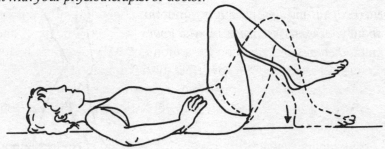

Lunge

Stand with feet apart in stepping position. Take weight forward on the front leg and bend at the knee and hip to lower your body toward the floor. Allow the back knee to bend and the heel of the back foot to lift off the floor.

NOTE: *If at any time you are uncertain about your exercises, discuss it with your physiotherapist or doctor.*

Vastus medialis obliquus retraining
Stand in a walk-stance position (as if you have just taken a step) with the front knee bent to 30 degrees and pull up the muscle on the inside of that knee. Arch the foot, then allow the foot arch to drop slightly. Repeat a number of times.

Alternatively, step down from a step and then back up, keeping the knee over the second toe.

NOTE: *If at any time you are uncertain about your exercises, discuss it with your physiotherapist or doctor.*

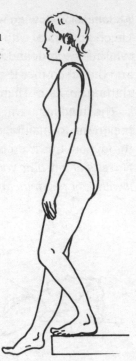

Hip extension with knee extension
Kneel on the mat on hands and knees with the pelvis and lower back in a neutral position. Straighten your left leg out behind you so that the knee is straight, and hold for 5 seconds. Slowly return to the kneeling position. Repeat with the right leg. It is important to maintain your pelvis and low back in a neutral position by using your abdominal muscles.

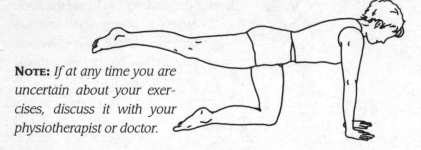

NOTE: *If at any time you are uncertain about your exercises, discuss it with your physiotherapist or doctor.*

Hip extension with knee bent

Kneel on the mat on hands and knees with the pelvis and lower back in a neutral position. Keep your left leg bent and take the sole of your foot toward the ceiling. Hold for 5 seconds. Slowly return to the kneeling position.

Repeat with the right leg. It is important to maintain your pelvis and low back in a neutral position by using your abdominal muscles.

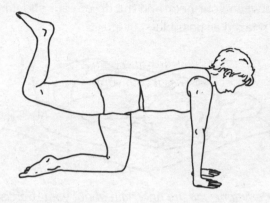

NOTE: *If at any time you are uncertain about your exercises, discuss it with your physiotherapist or doctor.*

Hip abductor strengthening

Lie on your side. Lock your knee straight, raise your leg and slowly bring it backwards. Hold for 3 seconds then slowly return. Keep your pelvis stable and maintain a true side-lying excessive hip hitching.

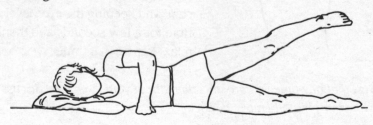

NOTE: *If at any time you are uncertain about your exercises, discuss it with your physiotherapist or doctor.*

Shoulder retraction with arm raise

Lie on your stomach with a rolled towel under your forehead, arms above your head, elbows slightly bent. Draw shoulderblade down and back in the direction of the opposite hip. Hold in that position and at the same time lift your arm 2–3 cm off the bed/floor. Lower your arm and relax, then repeat with the other shoulder. It is important to reduce the amount of activity in the muscle that is located between your neck and the tip of your shoulder. That is, keep it as relaxed as possible.

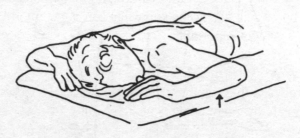

NOTE: *If at any time you are uncertain about your exercises, discuss it with your physiotherapist or doctor.*

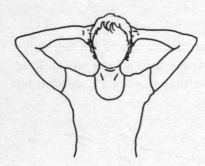

Neck retraction

Link hands behind the back of the head, well above the neck. Glide the head back without tilting it, giving yourself a 'double chin' and keeping the eyes level. Hold for a few seconds and then relax. Repeat 4–5 times.

NOTE: *If at any time you are uncertain about your exercises, discuss it with your physiotherapist or doctor.*

Take the example of Robert, who had had a back injury, a back operation and two falls over a period of five years. When he started his
exercise program, he was unable to lie on his back because of the pain.
He began with one 'repetition' of the abdominal hollowing exercise
because that was as long as he could tolerate lying on his back. By
working on his exercises each day he gradually increased the number
of repetitions he could manage. After two weeks, he was feeling much
more confident about being able to tolerate lying on his back.

So, it doesn't matter how many repetitions you start with.
Building up your confidence to know that you can do more despite
the pain is what is important.

Posture

Posture refers to the alignment of the body. In a way, we all know
what is meant by maintaining a 'good' posture. Most of us like to
lie about at home, often slouching on a sofa or armchair. Yet we
have all been told at one time or another that that sort of sitting is
'bad' for us. However, when you don't have pain it may not matter
very much if you have a poor posture, or sit in a poor posture for
a while. But if you do have pain, poor posture can make things
harder for you.

Don't get too carried away about posture, however. There really
is no perfect posture, and no one ever keeps a good posture all the
time. A general awareness of a good posture and an attempt to
maintain it as much as possible is usually enough for most people.

A 'good' posture is the correct alignment of the body so that all
the muscles can perform their required functions in the best possible way. Posture is not fixed and rigid. Every time we move or
remain in a sustained position, we are assuming some posture.
Ideally, that posture should be such that the muscles working
between the spine and the limbs can do the best job possible. If the
bony attachments are not in correct position because of poor posture, muscles will have to work at a mechanical disadvantage and
cause undue strain.

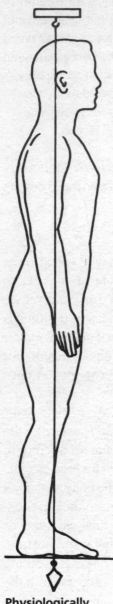

**Physiologically
Efficient Posture**

It can be easy to get into bad habits with our posture, especially if we are trying to favour one side or one part of our body because of pain. A common example is trying to walk with a small stone in your shoe. As a result, you may change the way you walk to accommodate the stone. If you continue in this altered posture you may eventually notice pain in the knee and hip. The diagram at left shows what the ideal standing posture would look like. While stretching and strengthening the muscles of the spine is important, it is also important that our spine muscles can hold the spine in a stable position. The lower part of the spine requires good stability in order to allow the hips, and in turn the legs to function properly. Likewise, the upper part of the body around the shoulderblades needs good stability to allow the shoulders and the arms to function properly and to relieve undue strain on the neck.

Take the example of Sally, who had been involved in an accident that had caused an injury to her neck. As a result of the length of time she had spent protecting and guarding her neck, she had developed changes to her posture.

Sally started using the stretch and strengthening exercises outlined in this chapter to improve her posture. In addition, rather than protecting and guarding her neck she tried to use it as normally as possible. She also started to use the other pain management coping strategies described in the following chapters. Gradually, Sally started feeling better about herself and was able to do things more confidently.

You can see this program is not a quick, or easy fix for your problems, but by persevering in the application of the strategies, you can regain much of your lifestyle. Of course you will have difficult times when you may feel it is not worth the effort. That is when you need to go over the pages in the book you have flagged as being important for you, and give yourself a little refresher course.

Lifting

One of the 'postures' that we assume throughout the day is the posture involved with lifting. Rather than practice a 'best' posture for lifting, it is more helpful to consider some general rules. First, wherever possible, avoid lifting by using mechanical aides as they can result in your developing or maintaining unhelpful postures. Second, if you must lift, reduce the weight. This may mean carrying two small bags of groceries from the car to the house rather than one heavy bag.

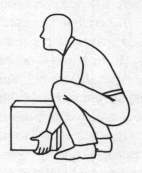

Raise the load so that you do not have to reach to the floor—for example, get your two year old to climb on the chair and lift her from that level. Hold the load close to your body. Get into a 'semi-squat' position with a small amount of bend in the knee, hip and trunk, not with the back fully bent forward (see the diagram on this page for an example of 'good' lifting).

Avoid twisting or bending sideways while lifting, and avoid lifting after periods of bending forward for a long time, such as after digging in the garden. Lift smoothly and slowly.

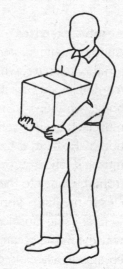

Safe Lifting and Carrying Positions

Preparing your body to be able to lift is of great importance. Strengthening the bones, ligaments and muscles by appropriate exercise is an essential part. Increasing the load you lift and the number of repetitions you lift by using the pacing principle of gradual increase will help prepare your body to perform the tasks safely.

One of the commonest triggers for back pain appears to happen when people are lifting. Naturally, people whose injury occurred while lifting are often very anxious about repeating this activity. The case of Robert (mentioned on page 139) provides a typical example.

Robert found it helpful to start lifting an empty box from the seat of a chair, and then gradually lowering the level until he was able to lift from the floor. At the same time, he started putting light weights into the box. Since one of his goals was to return to work, he started setting his lifting goals to try to reach a weight which was required for work.

He was not able to reach his pre-injury lifting goal, but he was confident of lifting lighter weights. This helped him to plan the type of work he could start considering. It has also helped him to accept that there would be some limits to the amount he could lift.

Aerobic exercises

Another name for aerobic exercise is cardiovascular or cardio-respiratory exercise, whicht means it is a way of exercising the heart (cardio), blood vessels (vascular) and lungs (respiratory) so that the body continues to use oxygen efficiently. The heart itself is a muscle. It needs exercise like other muscles in the body. The function of the heart is to pump blood through the blood vessels to the muscles, and return waste products. The blood carries oxygen from the lungs to the muscles, and carbon dioxide from the muscles to the lungs (from where it is expelled from the body).

Exercising muscles create a demand for more oxygen. The only way the muscles can get their supply of oxygen is for the person to breathe in more air, exercising the lungs, and then for the heart to pump it through the blood vessels, exercising the heart and blood vessels. If you become too puffed after exercise, then you are probably not getting enough oxygen (ie anaerobic exercise) and your body starts to build up too many acids. You can't keep this up for very long, especially if you are unfit.

The fitness of the heart can be measured by how fast it beats— that is, the pulse rate. A fit heart will give strong, slow contractions to pump the required volume of blood around the body. An unfit heart will give weak, rapid contractions in order to pump the same volume of blood around the body. As you get fitter, so will your heart.

Improved cardiovascular fitness will help to reduce feelings of tiredness and exhaustion. Getting fitter with aerobic exercise can also contribute to your sense of well-being. For exercise to be aerobic, it has to be performed continuously for 15–20 minutes 3–4 times per week with your heart rate within your training heart rate range. The range is calculated as 65–80 per cent of your maximum training heart rate range. Your maximum range is calculated at 220 minus your age. So, if you are 45 years old, your maximum range would be 220 minus 45, which equals 175.

Balance, coordination and skills acquisition

Good balance and coordination are a necessary part of the skills required to perform normal activities, as well as the more demanding skills often required in work places and sporting activities. Balance is a combination of muscle strength and flexibility, joint range of movement, messages being sent along the nervous system to the brain to help control the amount of muscle contraction to maintain balance, and the balance system in the brain.

In normal daily activities, we are using our balance system all the time. After a period of time when you are not moving as freely and as spontaneously as you used to, because of the pain, your balance becomes affected. The good news is that it is possible to retrain this balance system. To begin with, you can try holding on to a solid support you have confidence in while standing on one leg, and then alternating between legs. As you get better at this, try doing it without holding onto something. For more advanced work you should probably see a physiotherapist as he or she will probably have appropriate equipment.

Simon's case illustrates this point quite well. He had injured his back and shoulder and had been unable to resume playing golf. He identified this as one of his goals. So, along with his exercises he started practising some gentle chip shots with a practice golf ball. Over time, Simon's confidence improved and he developed a new posture to minimise the use of his shoulder while swinging the club. He started going to the driving range to practice his swing. Although he was not as competitive as he used to be, he found it extremely satisfying to be back playing his sport and socialising with his friends. He had come to terms with the fact that his handicap would be higher, but he realised that was not so important to him.

Maintenance and recording progress

Often the most difficult part of an exercise program is to keep it going. Have a look at Chapter 20 on maintaining your program. One of the important points is that initially you should discipline yourself to do your exercise program in a structured way every day. For example, you should set aside a specific time each day and ensure, as much as possible, that that time is always reserved for your exercise practice.

Ultimately, you could expect to reduce your exercises as you start replacing them with more of your functional tasks—that is, some of the goals you have set yourself. For example, if you have stairs at home or at work, then climbing those regularly could be built into your day. In that case you could leave extra stair climbing out of your exercise program. At the beginning, however, it is important to establish an exercise routine. Just remember that part of your exercise program is to help you become confident with moving.

One of the best ways to help you establish this routine is to record your progress each day in a type of diary or a chart. Write down or tick off each time you do your stretches, or how many repetitions of each exercise you have done. The strengthening exercise chart on page 132 is a good place to start this process.

Sports and chronic pain

If you want to resume some of your sporting activities you may have to consider what are realistic and achievable goals. Resuming your previous sports may not always be realistic, but you could consider resuming some form of sport. Bowls, bocce, boules and tenpin bowling are excellent examples of how you could use your lunging exercises. Obviously you would have to build up your grip strength to hold your bowl, but that could be included in your exercise goals. As you start focusing on more functional goals, it may become necessary to start setting new goals to help build up your tolerance for some new activities.

Can you think how it may be possible to return to golf? You understand your abdominal hollowing and your shoulderblade stability. When you assume your stance for golf, you would be aware of hollowing your abdominals to stabilise your lumbar spine, bending your hips and knees, keeping your upper body posture relaxed and having a relaxed grip of the club. The movement then should come from your hips and pelvis, with some movement of the feet. As you complete the backswing, the buckle of your belt should be facing away from the hole. As you allow the pelvis and hips to rotate 180 degrees, you end up with your buckle facing the hole. The club has just easily swung through to hit the ball sweetly onto the green. And all this has been done with your lumbar spine stable and your neck and shoulders relaxed.

Whichever realistically achievable sport you choose, the principle of setting baselines and pacing applies. For example, with your golf, to start, just do two or three short relaxed swings on the first day, then stop. Next day, attempt another few swings. Then calculate your average and take 80 per cent of that figure as your baseline. Then gradually upgrade your program to hit light practice balls and then progress to hitting actual golf balls. The important part is to progress slowly and steadily, not to feel that the only way to play is go out competitively for 18 holes. This is one of the hard things to do.

Susan was a perfect example of 'the typical golfer'. She suffered with neck pain and headaches that were restricting all aspects of her life. She was isolating herself, her marriage was failing and she lived in constant anxiety about getting to her chiropractor for an 'adjustment' every time she had a flare-up of pain. Susan was also a perfectionist. Her beliefs were that if she wasn't out playing competitive golf to attempt to reduce her handicap every game, then it wasn't worth playing. This was Susan's attitude when we first saw her. What she described was happening with her golf was that she was slamming the club through so hard that it hit the ground, sent a jolt through her neck and of course set up a pattern of pain with which she was unable to cope. Naturally, she stopped playing golf.

Susan attended the three-week ADAPT program at the hospital. By the end of the program, she had developed the confidence and knowledge to deal with the flare-ups in pain. She was using pacing, stretches, exercises and relaxation, as well as applying cognitive challenging to unhelpful thought patterns. She also started a few gentle golf swings, if somewhat skeptically to begin with. She was also able to manage her own flare-ups of pain without depending on her chiropractor to give her some short-term relief.

Susan came back to see us 12 months later. At this time she was relaxed and confident, she was enjoying a satisfying marriage and although she was seeing her chiropractor infrequently, she was not dependent on him to help her cope with her pain. When asked about her golf, she replied, 'I wouldn't have got out of bed 12 months ago for the kind of golf I am playing now'. What did Susan mean? She explained that she was enjoying her golf so much with a great group of women who also enjoy their golf, their lunches and the parties they organise.

Do you see what had changed? Her attitude. No longer was it so important to have the lowest score for the day, but the pleasure of the game was more important. Applying the program's strategies and thought challenging to her golf, along with the same simple tips given throughout this book had made a huge difference to Susan.

You will have noted that Susan was skeptical about her ability to return to golf. This is not an uncommon attitude for people starting out on this program of 'self-management'.

One of the pioneers in the field of pain management, clinical psychologist Professor Bill Fordyce at the University of Washington in the United States, once said that 'What matters is not what you thought at the beginning of a program like this, but rather what you think at the end'. Clearly, providing you are willing to give it a go despite your concerns, you are giving yourself a chance of managing your pain better.

Challenging Ways of Thinking About Pain

Persisting pain affects different people differently. For some, persisting pain can be extremely debilitating. For others, it is something they manage without much interference in their daily lives. While just about everyone with persisting pain gets distressed about it at times, they are not always distressed about it. So we have to ask, why do some find persisting pain disabling while others don't, and why do most people with such pain find it distressing at times but not other times.

One reason is that their pain is not always so bad. Generally, when pain is only mild it is not as troubling as when it is very severe. But research on chronic pain in a number of countries has also shown that the severity of pain is not the only reason people get troubled by it. There are often times when someone can have quite severe pain, but manage to not get distressed about it. Equally, it is possible to get distressed about pain even when it is quite mild. Look at a section of a letter we received from one of our former patients (we'll call her Jane).

Jane lived on a farm with her husband. Her persisting back pain had greatly limited what she could do around the farm. She was most concerned about not being able to ride her horses, either on the farm or in shows. During the time she participated in our programme she always stated that getting back on her horses was her main goal. We were more cautious and thought it would be too difficult (it would stir up her pain too much to be acceptable). After all, we believe that everyone with a chronic pain condition is likely to have some limits on what they can do. Accordingly, we encouraged her to think about less physically-demanding activities – ones which wouldn't aggravate her pain as much. But she stayed determined to do it.

During the programme Jane made good progress, paced up her exercises and ceased all her pain killers. Her mood also improved. She returned home to put her new skills into practice. She had a difficult time because her husband wasn't well and she had to help with many of the physically-demanding chores. But a year after leaving the programme she wrote to us to say:

> "we have been doing a little every day rather than all in a couple of days. I have to say that I feel as though I am thriving on it. I have been horse riding again, which I thought I would never be able to do, though it was my number one aim, and today was absolutely brilliant! Chasing bulls up and down hills, into and out of creeks and dams at full speed, on such a magnificent Autumn day, is what makes life worthwhile! My pain level was very high, especially afterwards, but hey, the day was great!
>
> Twelve months down the track, and it was a very hard track, I can move freely, easily, endure the pain much better and actually plan activities. Best of all, I can ride those beautiful horses and it feels as though there was no five year break!"

Jane still takes a little medication at times for her pain, but she described the amount *"as minute in comparison"* to what she used to take. At the same time, she described having *"a huge increase in my physical abilities"*.

What this shows is that despite doing something which did aggravate Jane's pain, she didn't become distressed. As she said, being able to ride again was worth more to her. She knew she wasn't causing herself any damage and that the increased pain after riding wouldn't last too long. She felt in control – after all, she knew that by riding her horse, especially in that vigorous way, she would make her pain worse, but she chose it. She also knew that if she paced the rest of her daily activities on the farm she could keep her pain under reasonable control – without relying on pain killers alone (as keeping her mind clear helped her to cope and to feel in control).

So that is a case of someone who is in a lot of pain but feeling happy. Earlier, before Jane attended the programme, she had been quite distressed when her pain was that severe. She was also much more disabled then and taking much more medication. When she first came to our clinic she was moderately depressed, but her pain ratings were no worse than they were when she was riding her horses.

So, by itself pain doesn't have to make us unhappy, frustrated, irritable and all the other negative feelings that often go with pain. You can check this yourself by keeping a small diary of your pain levels over a few days, along with a record of how you are feeling (happy, sad, frustrated, angry or whatever), the sorts of thoughts you are having at these times and the situation you are in (what you are doing or where you are). Copy out the recording sheet printed here into a notebook and carry it with you for a few days. Whenever you feel your pain is getting worse, stop what you are doing for a moment and write down:

(1) your **pain level** (on a 0-10 scale, where 0 = no pain and 10 = worst pain imaginable),

(2) the **thoughts you are having about your pain** (like "not again", "this is hopeless, I can't go on", "I must have overdone things, I'll just take it easy for a while", or whatever),

(3) **how you are feeling** (like happy, sad, angry, worried, or whatever). and

(4) **your situation** (what you are doing, or where you are, like driving the car, sitting at a desk, or whatever).

It is more helpful (and accurate) if you record your responses as close as possible to the time you feel your pain getting worse. If you leave it to the end of the day, your memory may not be as accurate.

We also recommend that you try not to read the rest of this chapter until you have made your own record of your responses to increased pain.

Try to make at least 10 entries in your diary, then have a look at what you have recorded.

Pain Response Diary

Date	Pain (0–10)	Thoughts (whatever is on your mind)	Feelings (happy, sad, etc.)	Situation (where, when)
Example	7	What's the use? Nothing works. I can't go on like this.	despair, hopeless	woken up, 2 am, in bed

Reviewing your diary

To begin with, look at the ways you have reacted (your feelings) and the pain levels at the time. Do you always react in the same way? Or does it change with different pain levels?

What else changes? Have a look at both your thoughts and the situations. Do you notice any links between your thoughts, your feelings, your pain and the situations you have been in? What might that suggest?

Now read the rest of this chapter. While you are reading it we would like you to think about your own pain and what you wrote in your pain response diary (as well as other times when your pain has been troubling or distressing you). It can help to discuss these issues with someone who knows you quite well as they may be able to act as a reasonably objective sounding board.

Helpful and unhelpful ways of thinking about pain

Remember the diagram in Chapter 1 (What is Chronic Pain?) of how chronic pain can lead to excessive suffering? If you can't recall it, turn back to Chapter 1 and have a look. One of the boxes in the diagram mentions unhelpful thoughts. You might have wondered what this meant. After all, many people who have chronic pain tell us that they think in negative ways **because** of their pain. They say that if their pain was relieved these negative thoughts would disappear too.

Negative reactions to pain appear quite normal responses. Some patients who come to our clinic tell us that anyone in pain would feel like that or think like that, and that if only we had pain we would feel like that too. No doubt there is some truth in these statements. But are they always true? Does it have to be like that? Do we have no choice in how we react to pain?

The story told by Jane shows us that we can be in a lot of pain but also be very happy and full of life. Another patient who attended our clinic can show us a different angle. This patient (we'll call him Joe) had previously had back surgery (a spinal fusion) and as that had not relieved his pain he later had a dorsal column stimulator implanted in his back. He told us that the electrical stimulation from this device had reduced the severity of his pain by 50%, but it was still about 5 out of 10. Despite this improvement, he continued to take strong pain killers (Opiates), he remained quite disabled at home, he was walking with the aid of a stick, and his mood was still very unhappy and often angry. He was especially angry about the unhelpful ways in which he felt he had been treated by his various doctors, his former employer and the workers compensation insurance company.

Joe was invited to attend our pain management programme. Initially, he was very skeptical. He couldn't see how it could help him. He felt he was doing as much as he reasonably could and if we weren't going to be able to take his pain away, then he couldn't see how the programme could help him. Still, he agreed to come. Although he had some difficult moments during the programme, when he had some heated disagreements with the staff (who he felt were not listening to him and were pushing him too much), he completed the whole three weeks. By the end of the programme, Joe said his pain was about the same as it had been before the programme, but he was doing many more exercises, he was walking without a stick, his mood was much more positive, he was much more confident that he could do things despite pain and he had stopped all his medication. He could even share jokes with the staff.

We have kept in touch with Joe since he left the programme and that is now over 4 years ago. He reports that he still has his pain, but it is a lot less (mostly only about 2 out of 10), he still uses his stimulator (but only for about 15 minutes a month), he hasn't taken pain killers on a regular basis for most of the last 4 years (and no opiates at all), his mood is generally very positive and stable (he is no longer easily angered), he keeps himself active around the house and he's doing a technical course with the aim of finding work again. Joe has even started playing golf again and he has taken up fishing again. By most measures we would say that Joe has successfully learned to manage his pain, and he would agree. Along with other graduates of ADAPT, he even comes to the clinic from time to time to talk to new patients about his experiences.

How did he do it? Well, to begin with Joe felt that unless his pain was relieved by at least 50% he would not be able to get back to a more normal lifestyle. After he had the stimulator implanted he found that even with 50% pain relief things weren't that much better. It was at that point that we talked to him about his role in managing his pain. Clearly, Joe couldn't rely totally on the stimulator to do it for him. One of the critical things he started to realise during our pain programme was that his reactions to his pain and to others were actually contributing to how he was feeling (his anger, his depression) and it was not just his pain that was doing it. Joe was also using his medication to block out his negative feelings, but they were also making him feel worse.

When we looked at Joe's pain response record in which he recorded his responses to increased pain we noted that when he was feeling distressed and angry, it was related more to his thoughts than to his pain. Thoughts like "this is hopeless", "I'll never get anywhere", I can't go on like this", "what's the point?" were usually linked to his distress and anger. His pain ratings went up and down, but his mood was worse when his thoughts were more negative and hopeless.

In other words, just as Jane had shown us earlier that aggravating your pain doesn't have to make you feel depressed, Joe has shown us that getting good pain reductions doesn't always mean we'll feel a lot better and be able to do a lot more. Both cases show us that how much pain affects us and what we do is strongly influenced by the ways we think about our pain.

Importantly, our thoughts are under our control. We can choose how we think. We might get into habitual ways of thinking at times, and we may feel we have no choice, but we can always change our minds.

With this realisation, Joe was encouraged to test out our method of improving his mood and changing the whole way his pain was interfering in his life. Despite his initial doubts, he has shown it is possible.

How did Jane and Joe do it?

(1) **First they came to see how the ways they thought about themselves, their pain and other people were playing a major role in how they felt and behaved.**

Thoughts are not just a running commentary on what you do – they play an active role in influencing your feelings and behaviour.

For instance, it is easy to react to activities which may cause more pain by thinking in a gloomy way. Instead of looking forward to seeing friends, or doing something enjoyable, you may find yourself dreading the travel involved, or the sitting or standing, and it may all feel too much effort when you have the pain to cope with as well.

These thoughts will probably make you feel more distressed than if you hadn't thought like that. Thinking like that may even make you change your mind, and give up the thing you had been looking forward to.

On the other hand, if you decided that the best way to deal with it was to "think positive" and ignore the pain you might just push ahead anyway, without planning, regardless of the consequences for yourself. But when your pain was aggravated, as is most likely, you could then say something like "see, I tried thinking positive and ignoring the pain and it didn't work". But is that the only way to look at what you did?

Or you might go, but be so worried about how you would feel by the end of it that you couldn't enjoy yourself. In this case, you might say "well I did it but I don't feel any better, so it was a waste of time". Again, is this the only way to look at what you did?

If you are starting to think "this doesn't apply to me", put it to the test. For the next few hours, tell yourself every few minutes: "there is no point in trying to manage my pain. I feel dreadful". How do you think you will end up feeling? If you don't think it will make any difference, why not try it? On the other hand, if you think it will make you feel worse, it will help you to see the possible effects of such thinking on your feelings.

Ways of thinking can also become habits, just like ways of doing things. And like other habits, some ways of thinking can become unhelpful. And like all habits, unhelpful thinking habits take an effort to change.

You may find it hard at first to see how you can change the ways you think and feel. Many people believe that they have no control over their thoughts and feelings – that they are just made like that. But in the past you must have thought things over to make a decision, or changed your mind about something, or kept your temper when you felt angry. How did it happen? Through hearing what other people said, perhaps, or thinking of the possible consequences of reacting in another way?

(2) The second important step is becoming a good listener to yourself

Most probably, you can recall having changed your mind about something after listening to yourself, and talking things through with yourself. This can also happen when you talk things over with someone else. Remember when you have explained a problem out loud, to someone who listens carefully, only to find that you solved it as you talked, and felt much more hopeful (and pleased with yourself!).

Getting things clear is often the start of feeling better and managing better. You can become a good listener to yourself.

(3) Identifying helpful versus unhelpful thoughts

Having a few worries and even a degree of unhappiness is a normal experience for all of us from time to time. But repeatedly becoming very worried or anxious or depressed for extended periods is not normal. In most instances we should be able to identify thoughts that are contributing to these more distressing emotions.

Often people describe their thinking at these times in terms of "positive" or "negative" thinking. These are terms most of us understand, but it often difficult to pin down exactly what they mean. As a result they can be misleading. For example, "thinking positively" can be OK at one level, when there are no major threats or problems. But when there is a major threat (like the development of a dark spot in your skin which could be a sign of skin cancer) simply thinking positively could result in your ignoring it and hoping it will go away. In this case, **positive thinking will not be helpful in sorting out the problem**. So thinking **too positively** can amount to denying that there is a problem. As a result you may not develop an effective plan to deal with a real problem. In the case of chronic pain, such thinking could result in your overdoing things and making your pain worse than it needs to be. **Positive thinking may help to keep your spirits up, but it is not usually enough for good problem solving.**

Negative thinking is similar to positive thinking in that it could be quite inaccurate, but in the opposite direction. So thinking negatively could mean that you think nothing will ever be any better. Such thoughts are likely to be obstacles to your even trying to have a go at doing something.

Of course, there are often a number of ways to look at most situations. There's a common saying that there are always two sides to every story. In fact, there could be more than two sides. So, there are often many ways in which you can deal with a problem, but some will be more effective than others.

Rather than talk in terms of "positive" or "negative" thinking when trying to deal with real problems like living with pain, it can be more useful to talk about "helpful" versus "unhelpful" thinking.

Helpful ways of thinking are those which enable you to deal effectively with a problem or source of stress. Helpful thinking may not solve all problems, but it should allow you to make some progress. In contrast, unhelpful ways of thinking are those which cause you even more distress. Unhelpful thinking may be understandable, but not helpful. For instance, when you are in a lot of pain it would be understandable and even accurate if you were to think your situation was terrible and completely unfair. But would it help if it led you to feel even more distressed? On the other hand, it might be more helpful if you were to acknowledge that your pain was severe, but at the same time to say to yourself that the best way for you to deal with it is to stay as calm as possible and avoid extreme reactions, reminding yourself that you've had pain like this before and you know it will pass and you will be OK. Such thinking could help you to minimise your level of distress and to feel more in control.

Helpful thinking doesn't mean telling yourself you are not in pain or that you don't have any problems. That might be called "positive thinking", but it is only denying real problems and while it might buy temporary comfort, you can't kid yourself forever.

As a rule, helpful thinking will be reasonably accurate. You will usually deal with a problem more effectively if you can assess it accurately. Accurate assessment can allow you to prepare for a challenge or stress appropriately. Overly positive assessments of problems risk underestimating the size of the task facing you. Equally, overly negative assessments risk overestimating the size of the task.

So, if you find yourself becoming increasingly agitated over your pain spend a few moments checking on your thoughts. Are they helping you to cope or are they making you feel more distressed? If they aren't helping, even if you feel they are justified, they must be challenged.

Here are two examples of how common reactions to pain can build into major self-defeating events if left unchecked.

(1) When worry grows into anxiety and then panic

We all worry at times – in fact, a little worry helps to keep us safe from taking unwise risks. But when it goes on and on, and leads to unwise decisions, it's no help at all. The following diagram shows the sort of vicious circle that can develop.

For example: Think of being in a difficult situation, such as at a crowded supermarket or in a car on a busy road, and you feel your pain is getting worse. . . .

What if your reactions were like these?

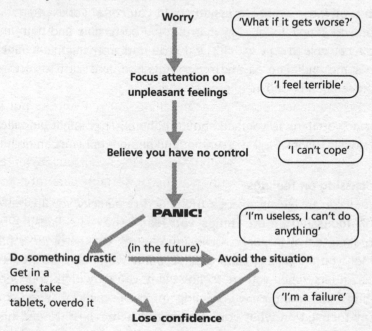

Try following the arrows through, remembering the last time you got into difficulties when your pain flared up. These are common reactions, but there are other ways of reacting the are more helpful.

In general, people get panicky when:

- they believe the threat or possible harm is greater/worse than it is,
- they think they are very likely to come to harm,
- and they forget how they can cope.

So, at times of difficulty with your pain, you need to check –

(1) Are you being realistic about the risk? For instance, if your pain is increasing, how likely is it that it will become unbearable and lead to something awful? (how often has it really got like that before?)

(2) even if the worst happened could you cope? For example, do you find yourself worrying that it could be terrible and that you won't be able to cope with it? Or do you start worrying that it might be some undiagnosed and serious disease, and start to picture yourself bed-bound, helpless, or worse?

Or do you think to yourself about all the other possible (and less serious) reasons for it worsening, and about what you can do?

Focussing on feelings

When you are feeling anxious, frightened, or panicky, you are probably **focussing on the things you fear** – such as collapsing, or breaking down in public, or losing control. On the other hand, when you are feeling calm, you probably won't be thinking like this. In fact, when you are feeling calm, you may think you were being "silly" when you were feeling anxious or panicky. **When you stay focused on what you're trying to achieve or do and not how you feel**, you are more likely to feel calmer.

To help you see how your thinking can affect your feelings, try the following exercise:
Think of an anxiety-provoking situation that you have experienced with your pain. Replay that situation in your head – from start to finish – to recall the fears you felt at the time. Then – staying calm – try to work out how likely those fears were. (For example, would you really have collapsed? And even if you did, would no one have helped?). It is also quite likely you would have coped successfully before with this sort of situation. Look at the effect of reminding yourself of that.

Your **confidence** is also important when it comes to dealing with fears and worries. Unfortunately, you can't just get confidence without any effort. What other people say can make you feel more or less confident about how you cope. But what you say to yourself will make the biggest difference. When things go badly, do you criticise yourself? Do you tell yourself you are "useless", "hopeless" or "stupid"? If so, stop and ask yourself. . . .

Am I being fair to myself?
Is it helpful to think like this?

The answer to both is – **NO**. This sort of thinking is undermining you. Imagine how you would feel if someone else said it to you.

To think about it another way. When you do something well, how often do you tell yourself you are "clever", "brilliant" or "capable". Most people say they don't do this, but they are quite prepared to say very negative and critical things to themselves when they make a mistake. If you treated someone else in this way, say your children or friends or even your dog, what might be the result? So why do it to yourself?

Remember the example of the leading sports players that we see on TV. When they do something well, whether it is a fast time, a good kick or they save a goal, they usually show how pleased they are – they recognise their achievements. Equally when they make a mistake they try to work out where they went wrong and how to do it better next time. The successful players don't waste time getting into a stew over their mistakes – they try to learn from them and avoid repeating them.

The same methods can be used in coping with pain.

Confidence comes from doing things as well as possible – recognising it yourself – and remembering it – and telling yourself (and even other people) about it.
Coping with your pain, and carrying on as normal a life as possible despite it, are things you know how to do well. When you feel your pain getting stirred up, stopping to think and plan your next step instead of panicking is a success in itself. If you expect

yourself to manage perfectly, you will rarely be satisfied. If you are realistic about what you can manage, and achieve it, or get some way towards it, you have every right to be pleased. And when you are pleased with your achievements, you will gain confidence.

So how about undoing the vicious circle to make it look like this:

When you start to:

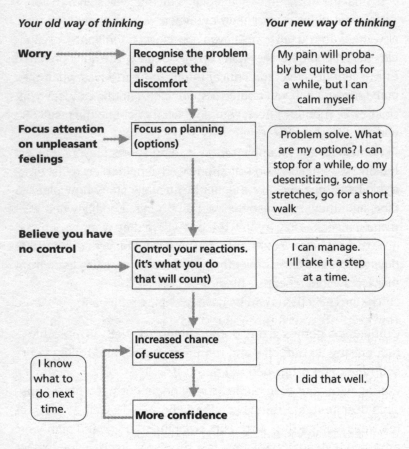

More Helpful Reactions to Increased Pain

Your old way of thinking   *Your new way of thinking*

Worry ─────────► Recognise the problem and accept the discomfort

My pain will probably be quite bad for a while, but I can calm myself

Focus attention on unpleasant feelings ───► Focus on planning (options)

Problem solve. What are my options? I can stop for a while, do my desensitizing, some stretches, go for a short walk

Believe you have no control ─────► Control your reactions. (it's what you do that will count)

I can manage. I'll take it a step at a time.

Increased chance of success

I did that well.

I know what to do next time.

More confidence

Try these methods out on yourself. You may find it useful to start by remembering a recent occasion when you had difficulty coping with your pain. Think about how you managed it then and how you might manage it now using the methods outlined here. When you feel your pain is starting to bother you again try these methods out and then review how you managed. What can you learn from your first attempts? How could you do it better?

If you are finding it difficult to master by yourself, it may be helpful to work on these methods over a few sessions with a clinical psychologist. They are specially trained to help people in this way.

(2) Accepting that your pain could last a long time
No one wants to live with pain. Coming to terms with having chronic pain and accepting you may have to live with it for a long time is hard for everyone who has it. If your doctor says there's no cure for your pain and "you will just have to learn to live with it" he or she may not tell you how to do that. You might think "well it's all very well for him or her, they don't have pain". You are also likely to refuse to believe your doctor is right – maybe if you keep looking you will eventually find a doctor who can fix you. You may think something like "after all, 'they' can transplant hearts and kidneys and do all sorts of wonderful things, so surely 'they' can fix my pain?"

Possibly because of all the news and information we get these days it often seems that we have come to almost expect all health problems to be solved or be close to it. Almost daily we hear of "breakthroughs" in the fight against some disease or other. However, if you keep listening you will also often hear that the study was done on rats in a laboratory and it may be 5 years or more before the new treatment will be available to humans.

For some time you are likely to view your pain as "acute". You will say to yourself things like "it's only been a short time since I got it and it's bound to settle soon". But those weeks can become months then years. It is true that pain conditions like back pain usually wax and wane over time, but for many people it never goes away for long. For others, some pain will be present most of the time but every now and then it will get worse for a period. Over time, the periods when it is worse may become more frequent. If you keep waiting for the pain to go away, or for someone to take it away for you, it is likely that you will have a long wait. In the meantime, what is happening to your life? Your family? Your work? Your friends?

Recognising these effects is an important part of coming to terms with your pain. It can help you to start problem-solving and stop waiting for something to happen.

It is likely that you will have tried try to keep up most or all of your normal activities – at home, at work, in your sport or social life. But if these activities make your pain worse you are likely to start finding many of these activities become disrupted by the pain. Some will push on regardless and suffer more pain as a result, as we discussed in the chapter on pacing. Others will stop what they are doing and may start to avoid many activities which aggravate their pain. At these times you may say to yourself things like, "I'll take it easy for a while and things might improve". You may even get advice from your doctor or physiotherapist to "let pain be your guide" – or whenever you do something which makes your pain worse, stop that activity. That can be acceptable for a few minor tasks, especially if there's someone else to do it for you and you never really liked doing it anyway, like washing the dishes or doing the grocery shopping.

However, as we discussed in the chapter on the effects of pain on your lifestyle, cutting back on normal daily activities can lead to deconditioning of your body and to your putting on more weight. This, in turn, can lead to more pain. It can also lead to frustration, especially if you start to think about all the things you have given up or can't do as well as you used to. In fact, not being able to do something you would really like to do, especially if it is due to pain and that pain was due to something that was not your fault, can lead to a great deal of frustration. Over time, it can lead to resentment. You may wonder what you've done to deserve this. Some people us that they feel it is almost as if they are being punished for something.

When you keep trying to put the pain to oneside and to get on with your life, but you keep having set-backs and feel you are not getting anywhere, you might also start to feel hopeless or despondent. You may feel that you will never get on top of it.

Equally, when you repeatedly get your hopes up about a new treatment or seeing a new doctor or clinic, only to have them dashed, it is likely you will start to feel helpless or even desperate. Many patients at our clinic tell us that they are prepared to "try anything". To us it often seems that people with chronic pain who keep seeking treatments which keep failing are like people who have been unemployed a long time and have had repeated knock-backs from prospective employers. And, of course many people with chronic pain are unemployed and that will often make their problems even worse. After having these sorts of experiences for a while, it is not surprising that many people with chronic pain start to feel helpless and depressed. Eventually they may feel despair at the prospects of anything ever improving again. Some may feel that life is not worth living anymore.

The despair that can come with repeated treatment failures is often coupled with a sense of loss. The sense of loss is usually to do with having had to give up activities that were enjoyable and gave life some of its meaning, such as work, sport or just going fishing. The sense of loss can also be related to loss of feeling well and healthy or robust. In some ways, aspects of loss for people with persisting pain can be like the loss that we all feel as we age and can no longer do the things we used to do or no longer look so young and fresh. Yet we often hear people saying that they would like to grow old gracefully. That means accepting that you are getting older and seeking out the opportunities that aging can provide. In contrast, others refuse to acknowledge they are aging and seek to appear as young as possible, often doing the things they couldn't afford to do when they were young.

If you find yourself getting into these situations, what are your options?

Well, it can help to talk such feelings through, with yourself or with someone else, to get a more balanced view. One of the difficulties is that the memory plays tricks when you are depressed. This can make it easier to remember unhappy events and the times when you have not coped, and harder to remember much about times when you have managed well. This means you have to make an extra effort to think it through clearly.

It is important to realise that some sadness at times (but not all the time) is a normal reaction to having persisting pain. After all, no one usually wants to live with pain. So try not to be too hard on yourself if you do feel a little low at times. However, if you find yourself starting to feel low for much of the time and you're having trouble pulling yourself out of it, then it probably is time to do something about it.

It can help to write down your thoughts, and your feelings, especially when you are feeling a bit gloomy or your pain is getting worse. Try to see where these thoughts and feelings lead.

For instance, you may be looking around at the house or garden . . . you notice something that needs doing . . . then you think about the difficulties of doing it . . . and about the increased pain it could cause . . . and you start to tell yourself that things around the house are getting in a state . . . you couldn't ask anyone round because of it but you can't go out to see friends because of the pain . . . so you won't see anyone . . . you'll be trapped indoors getting frustrated at it all . . . it hardly seems worth getting up in the morning . . . what is there to look forward to, and so on.

What started with noticing a job which needed doing has quickly led downhill to feeling that life is hardly worth living – and this can happen in a few seconds. In fact, you may well not be aware of the thoughts, just of the feeling of complete hopelessness, and it will seem as if it came out of the blue. But it didn't come out of the blue. **Your thoughts led you to that point**, and the best way to begin to catch these streams of thoughts is to write them down, and to think about them. That is the first step to being able to stop them, and to stop yourself from feeling like that. After all, if you read back through the thoughts, they are not the whole picture. What you should be aiming for is **realistic, helpful thinking**.

It is harder to do this when you are feeling extremely distressed. It is much easier to catch yourself slipping – starting to think in unhelpful and increasingly desperate ways – early. If you wait until you feel extremely hopeless before you try to drag yourself out of it, it will usually be much harder than if you'd stopped yourself getting to that point.

If you find yourself repeatedly getting frustrated or depressed about your pain there are some relatively simple steps you can take to get things back into balance.

(a) First you need to **identify the sorts of thoughts** you have at these times.

(b) Then you need to **examine them carefully**, and see if they are a fair picture.

Remember that it can be hard to remember the more positive things in life (including your own strengths and qualities).

Start early: it's much harder to tackle the despair at the end of the line than the partial picture at the beginning.

Taking the example given above, you could **ask yourself questions like**:

. . . does this job I have noticed really need doing? . . . is it urgent? . . . am I the best person to do it? . . . What about help from others? . . . if I am going to do it (with or without help), does it have to lead to increased pain? . . . What about pacing, or preparing by doing some stretch exercises, planning how you could do it, and so on? . . . Is it really a higher priority than me? . . . if it's not done, is it really true that the house is not fit to have friends in? . . . What sort of friends judge you by the state of your house? . . . Do you judge others like that? . . . and so on.

At each point, you need to ask yourself how realistic the thoughts are, and whether they are helpful. It can also be useful to remind yourself of how you have coped in the past, and how you learned to cope with your pain at times. Think about how you would help someone else who was thinking and feeling like this – would you be telling them that life was not worth living? (so why tell yourself things like that?)

What all this adds up to is **REALISTIC AND HELPFUL THINKING**.

Unrealistic and unhelpful thinking can be all negative, like the examples above. Or it can be expecting too much of yourself, setting such high standards that you will never reach them.

It can be helpful to ask yourself things like:

> "What is the worst that can happen?"
> "Would it be so awful that I couldn't cope at all?"
> "How likely is it anyway?"
> "How might you deal with it if it did happen?"

Once you have answered these sorts of questions, you will be in a good position to handle even the worst situation.

Unrealistic thinking can also be too positive, denying that there is any problem, and setting you up for overdoing and failure.

After all, if someone else tells you to "cheer up and forget about the pain", you probably, quite rightly, feel angry and misunderstood.

Ignoring your pain as much as possible and trying to act as if it wasn't there can work for a while. But in the end you won't be able to kid yourself about it forever.

For example, one lady who came to our clinic told us that during the week she tried to keep herself as busy as possible at work and at home. This helped her to not notice her pain for much of the time. But often on the weekends when she was trying to relax she found her pain was worse than ever. When she tried to pace her activities more effectively during the week, she found she had less pain on the weekend. This meant that by acknowledging her pain she was able to develop ways to get around it. Whereas before she had denied the existence of the pain and paid the price of that each weekend.

While it doesn't help to think about your pain all the time, it also doesn't help – or not for long – to simply tell yourself just to get on with it and forget the pain. Pain patients often talk about "fighting the pain". But who can win, when the pain is yours? Who loses? How long can you keep this battle up?

Perhaps it would be more effective to use your strength to negotiate with the pain over what you can do, and how you will do it.

Helpful, realistic thinking is accurate, balanced, and gets things in perspective – not just looking at the problems, but also about the resources you bring to the problem: a good brain, ways of managing pain, and a reasonably fit body.

Helpful thinking means that you are as clear as you can be about your limits, but they don't overshadow all that you can do within them. It means that you appreciate your past successes, and that gives you confidence for the future. It means that you can ask friends or family members for help which they can give, and offer appreciation and perhaps another sort of help in exchange.

Remember, these ways of thinking are all habits. They are not easy to change – but they can be changed. And they won't change on their own, nor will tablets take them away. In fact, people who take tablets to calm them down, or brighten them up, tend to believe it's the tablets working when they feel better, but blame themselves when they feel worse – so there's no way to win with this approach!

You may think that this is all a bit unnecessary – like icing on the cake. But years of helping chronic pain patients to change their lives has shown that working on the way you deal with your thoughts and feelings is as important as working on exercises.

Making changes, getting fit, feeling better and achieving more doesn't last unless you recognise that it is due to your efforts – not just the doctor or physiotherapist you have been seeing. After all, if you put all your improvements down to others, it would make it hard for you to keep going when they weren't around.

Some points to remember:

- When you are not managing so well, try to remind yourself that you have the means to get back on course – by challenging the worries or the hopelessness, and changing them.
- If you put your successes down to chance, it will be harder to make steady gains, and to look forward to what you can make of your life.
- If you are too hard on yourself when you make mistakes or if you set such high standards that you are bound to fail, progress will be that much harder

Challenging unhelpful thoughts

When you are aware of feeling irritable, anxious, hopeless, or miserable . . . **stop and listen to what you've been saying to yourself**. Try writing it down (use the recording form shown earlier in this chapter). Read through the examples in this chapter, and use the questions suggested. You may find yourself feeling a certain way at particular times – maybe when you can't sleep, or before exercise, or when you are bored with what you're doing.

When you are ready, have a look at what you've written. Ask yourself about the thought:

"Is that a fair judgement or statement?" and
"Is it helpful to think like that?"

You could also ask yourself:

"Are there other ways, more helpful ways, I could look at this?"

Underneath your initial, unhelpful thoughts write down the answers to these questions, or anything else that helps you to get things in perspective. Also write down any feelings associated with these new thoughts.

For example,
One patient who attended our programme wrote that when he had thoughts like "this is hopeless" "I can't go on" "The pain's unbearable", he felt depressed, hopeless.

Then he challenged these thoughts by saying things like:

"well I've had pain like this before and I have managed" "I know I'll be OK, I haven't injured myself again, so it will settle". "I'll work out a plan to get through the next little while" "I'll take a step at a time, cut back on the more vigorous activities, but keep doing things I can manage"; "the pain is quite bad, but it's been like this before and I know it will settle sooner or later". When he had thoughts like these he reported starting to feel back in control again.

Of course, he had to keep doing it. But that's no different to cleaning your teeth. We all know that if we stop cleaning our teeth we are likely to have trouble with them. So we take care of our teeth and prevent problems by taking a few minutes each day to clean them. The same approach can apply to managing chronic pain.

If you keep checking for unhelpful thoughts and reactions to pain, and challenging those thoughts when you spot them, your mood will be under your control much more (rather than being controlled by your pain).

With practice, it get easier. Remember how learning to drive, or cook, or sew or do carpentry seemed almost impossible at first – and still look pretty complicated to those who can't do them. They took lots of concentration and practice. You would also have tried to learn from the inevitable mistakes you made. But after a while, you could drive or cook while you talked, or listened to the radio, even though you were making complex decisions very rapidly in order to do so. Challenging and changing your unhelpful thoughts is just the same. It can become a very useful habit. The key is to recognise the unhelpful thoughts as soon as they appear – don't wait until you are really down in the dumps before you start to challenge them.

We should emphasise that challenging unhelpful thoughts doesn't mean trying to stamp them out or just blocking them – if you try these techniques you'll find they keep coming back. Instead, challenging unhelpful thoughts means identifying other, more helpful ways to look at things and moving on with those. The unhelpful thoughts can be left to the side and you don't need to waste energy on them.

Further reading

If you would like to read more about this way of dealing with emotional problems we would recommend that you find "Beating the Blues", by Susan Tanner and Jill Ball, two clinical psychologists from Sydney.

If reading this book or others like it is not enough, then we would recommend that you ask you local doctor to recommend a psychiatrist or clinical psychologist with expertise in this area. If persisting pain is the main problem then we would recommend that your doctor refer you to a nearby multidisciplinary pain clinic or centre for a full assessment.

12

Using Relaxation

Relaxation is a feeling of being calm. In some situations you may feel drowsy when you are relaxed, especially if you are feeling tired. At these times, relaxation can help you go off to sleep. On the other hand, there are times when you can be wide awake, alert and relaxed, as for example, when you are concentrating calmly on something. At these times, relaxation can help you to concentrate better, without getting too tense and distracted.

The ability to relax can be very helpful whether or not you have a pain problem. When you do have a pain problem, relaxation is that much more important. It is important for a number of reasons:

- **Relaxation can help to reduce tension and to stop pain getting worse.** Getting wound up or tense doesn't cause chronic pain, but it will often make pain worse. This can lead to a vicious cycle of pain— tension—more pain—more tension.

- **Relaxation will help you to calm yourself and to feel more in control despite the pain and other stresses.** Pain will often result in distress, irritability, and feelings of helplessness. All these feelings make it harder to cope with pain.

- **Relaxation can help you to get to sleep.** Getting to sleep when you have pain can be difficult. If you wake up during the night, pain can make it hard to get back to sleep.

Of course, for many people, being able to relax is easier said than done. That is one reason why so many people use tranquillisers and sleeping tablets. But these tablets are really meant for short-term use only. In other words, they are not suitable for people with chronic pain in the long run. Learning to relax is not only better for you, it is also more helpful than long-term use of these tablets.

Relaxation makes you feel good. It has no unpleasant side effects. It helps you to sleep naturally—with no hangovers. The more you use relaxation, the more effective it will be.

Even though you may have found it difficult to relax in the past, that doesn't mean it's impossible. It simply means that you'll have to learn how to do it better and you will have to put aside quite a bit of time to practise it.

Relaxation is really just a skill. Just as driving a car, playing bowls, cooking and speaking a foreign language are skills. No one is born with these skills—we all learn them. To become proficient at these skills you have to practise them. The same goes for relaxation. The actual way you relax doesn't really matter, just as long as you do it when you need to.

Try to relax:
- When you feel yourself getting tense or irritable
- When you feel the pain is getting worse
- When you want to get to sleep

At ADAPT we use a relaxation technique that you can use anywhere, once you are good at it. If you already have your own technique and you are happy with it, keep using it. You may already have your own way of relaxing, such as having a nice long bath or sitting on a park bench and watching the world go by. This, of course, just shows that even if you feel you can't relax there are times when you have relaxed. Perhaps you could build on these experiences and get into the same frame of mind at other times?

It is important that you practise relaxing in different places, not just lying on your bed or on the floor. This is because your pain can get worse anywhere and you won't always be able to lie down at those times or places. If you relax by reading, watching TV or going for a quiet walk, that is also fine and you should keep doing them. But you won't always be able to do those things when you need to relax. So it's important for you to learn a relaxation exercise that you can do anywhere.

How to relax

To begin with, you should practise in a sitting or lying position. As you get better at it you should try relaxing when you are standing, walking and even while you are doing other things, like talking and driving. You may feel you have too much on your mind or no time to relax. If so, it will help if you give yourself 'permission' to set aside some time to relax. You can come back to those things on your mind afterwards, and your mind might be clearer then.

Step 1
- Make yourself as comfortable as possible. You may close your eyes, but you don't have to.
- Take a deep breath, hold it a moment and then let it out slowly.
- Let yourself go loose and floppy as you breathe out.
- When you are ready, take another deep breath and let that go slowly.
- Now let your breathing return to normal. Don't go on deep breathing. This first part is just to loosen you up.

Step 2
- Keep in mind that you must not force yourself to relax, that will only make you more tense.
- Let yourself relax by letting go the tension in your muscles each time you breathe out.
- Imagine that each time you breathe out, the tension is draining away from your body. Even if you think it isn't, try to imagine it is.

Step 3

Try to keep your mind off the pain and other worries. There are many ways to do this. Here are a few:

- Repeat one or more words over and over in your mind. Do it slowly and without forcing it. For example, you could repeat the words 'one' or 'relax' or 'calm'.
- Imagine a relaxing, peaceful or happy scene in your mind, such as a holiday you once had, or one you would like to have.
- Keep your eyes open and focus on a particular part of the room or wherever you are. Keep staring at the spot in a calm, fixed way.

Your mind will still wander, especially to begin with. When you notice it has wandered, gently bring it back to what you were doing. Try not to get annoyed about it, just be patient. Within a week or so this will get easier.

Basically, that's all there is to it. There are three important points to keep in mind:

1 Make time to practise, but don't try to relax (don't force it).
2 Let your muscles go loose each time you breathe out.
3 When your mind wanders, gently bring it back to the task.

Practice makes perfect

As with all skills, the only way to become good at relaxing is to practise it as often as possible. To begin with, practise this relaxation technique at least seven times a day. These practice sessions should include two long sessions (15–20 minutes each) and five short sessions. The short sessions may be anything from 30 seconds to 5 minutes in length. Most importantly, the short sessions should be done in different places throughout the day. Practise the long sessions in a place that is quiet or where you won't be disturbed. But you should practise the short sessions in all sorts of places, even if they are noisy. If you practise relaxing in one place only, you will find it harder to do it in other places. But if you practise relaxing wherever and whenever you get a moment, you will get better and better at doing it anywhere.

Of course, it is often easier to relax in places that are quiet—but these are not usually the places where you get tense. So, even though it may be more difficult in some places, you should still practise relaxation techniques there. Before long you will notice you are getting better at it.

To help you get into a routine of regular relaxation practice, make a copy of the Relaxation Practice Chart below. Each time you complete a session, tick it off on the chart. Before long, you will find practising is starting to become a habit and you won't need to continue filling in the chart.

Applications of relaxation

Relaxation Practice Chart

Date	20 min	20 min	5 min	5 min	5 min	5 min	5 min

- **Be realistic in your expectations.** It will take time to become good at relaxing in difficult circumstances. You may never achieve the level of relaxation you would like, but it will help if you can just take the edge off your tension.
- **Get in early.** Don't wait until you are feeling really tense or upset before trying to relax. It is much easier to relax when you first start to feel the tension rising.
- **Check your level of tension wherever you are.** If you're sitting or standing on a bus or train, or while your car is stopped at the traffic lights, check for signs of tension. It may be a clenched jaw, a tight neck, or the whites of your knuckles while you're holding the steering wheel of your car. If you notice any tension, start relaxing.
- **Relax while you are doing other things.** If you can't stop what you are doing, just try to work on letting the tension go each

time you breathe out. In this way you can relax while you are talking, walking, or even when you are driving your car. It doesn't matter if you can't 'switch off', letting go the tension is the important thing.

- **Be ready to relax as often as you need to.** Even though you did your relaxation practice in the morning, this won't stop you from getting tense in the afternoon. If it is a stressful day, you may need to use your relaxation technique many times that day. On the other hand, if it's a relaxing day you may not need to use your technique at all.

Attentional Techniques – Distraction and Desensitising

13

Summary:

- Many people use distraction to cope with their pain.
- But distraction is only one of many possible mental techniques that involve using your attention. We call them attentional techniques as a group.
- They won't remove the pain completely, but they can take the edge off it.
- Combining desensitising with other activities can help you to keep active.
- We recommend you should apply them <u>whenever</u> you feel your pain is starting to bother you.
- Three strategies are outlined, but they all need practice to develop into useful tools.
- Try each one to work out which suit you best; you may find one suits better in one situation while another suits you better in other situations.

1. Focus your attention away from the pain (Distraction)

These techniques work best if you can involve as many of your senses as possible. This means using your senses of sight, hearing, smell, temperature and touch, all at once. By really getting involved in this way you will find it easier to block out the pain signals.

- **Imagine a pleasant, relaxing scene.** Imagine you are really there. Focus on what you can see, hear, smell and feel – the colours around you; the sound of the sea, or birds; the warmth of the grass or sand under your body, and so on. It may be a favourite place, by the sea, in the countryside or in your garden. If it was a time or place you associate with happy feelings, try to recall those too. But make sure you don't start to focus on any sad feelings, such as dwelling on how unhappy you have been since that time or how you can't go back to those days.

- **Plan something you can look forward to**, such as a holiday, changes to your house or garden, or an evening entertaining friends. Dwell on the pleasant aspects, and expand on all the details. Make it as real as possible.

- **Bring to mind someone important to you**, perhaps a member of your family or a friend whom you would very much like to see. Make a clear picture of him or her in your mind's eye, and imagine you're having a chat. [Make sure you do not start talking about pain!]

- **Focus your mind on something you can see**, using it to block out awareness of anything else. It could be a pain-free part of your body, a picture on the wall, other people around you, the scene outside your window.

- **Try recalling the plot and characters, in a favourite book** or one you are reading at present. Build up as much detail as you can manage.

- **Recite poetry, or a song** – one you particularly enjoy, and is calming.

You may have some distraction ideas of your own. Try them too.

2. Imagine Scenes Which Include The Pain, But Focus On Pleasant Or Exciting Aspects Of The Scene.

• Create an **exciting and inspiring scene** in which you are over-riding your pain in order to achieve a greater goal – running the last stretch of the marathon, winning a tennis match, scoring a goal in a football final, or getting to the top of Mt Everest without oxygen.

3. Focus on the Pain Itself (to desensitise yourself to your pain)

At first glance this technique may seem to go against 'common sense' as it involves letting yourself feel the pain rather than trying to get away from it. To help it make more sense, think about why we get pain to start with. Broadly speaking, acute pain is a warning signal. It warns us that something is wrong, we may have an injury or be about to have an injury. Acute pain lets us know we need to investigate the cause and do something about it. Such pain can be useful to us. But that does not apply to chronic pain.

In contrast, with chronic pain any damage has already been done, so it's not really telling us anything new. The possible cause of your chronic pain will have been extensively investigated and you should have been reassured that serious or life-threatening causes have been ruled out. You can tell yourself that you are physically OK and not in danger.

Earlier in the book we mentioned that one of the main mechanisms involved in chronic pain is a process called Central Sensitisation. This means that harmless nerve signals can be experienced as pain. The trouble is, our brain may still see the pain as a threat, just like acute pain. Unfortunately, just telling yourself the pain is OK is unlikely to be enough to overcome chronic pain. We have found that you also need to <u>train</u> your brain to learn not to react to this chronic pain as if it is acute pain.

How do we train our brain to learn this new skill? Just like any other training – by practising it (a lot).

To desensitise yourself to your chronic pain you need to:

1. Accept that it is not harmful and that it is OK to start moving.
2. Try not protecting yourself against the pain.
3. Acknowledge the pain is there but don't react to it.

This requires that you don't try to avoid or escape the pain. The normal response to ongoing pain is to try to get away from it or to distract yourself from it – that is why people take pain killers. But what would happen if you didn't try to get away from it? Remember, you'll have the pain anyway. Why not see what happens if you don't try to escape the pain?

Another way of looking at our response of trying to avoid or escape from pain is to compare it with what we might do when we are afraid of something that is not really dangerous. For example, if we have a fear of heights we might avoid going to high places, even though it is very unlikely that we would fall off. By avoiding heights, we may never learn that we'd be OK after all. That fear can also limit our lifestyle. Interestingly, we know that the best treatment for these sorts of fears is confronting whatever you are afraid of (like going up to a high place) and letting yourself feel the anxiety sensations without reacting. It may take a few sessions of repeating this, but if you keep at it consistently, the method will work and you will overcome the fear. This effect can be called desensitisation or habituation (getting used to something).

Habituation is something we have all experienced. For example, if you buy a new painting or poster and put it on your wall you will notice it and admire it whenever you walk past initially. But after a few weeks you notice it less. It will start to become part of the background. You remain aware that it is there, you just don't notice it as much. This effect is called habituation. If we weren't able to do it we would be constantly distracted by everything we walked past. To become habituated to something we must not try to avoid or escape from it. Repeatedly trying to escape from or avoid something keeps us more sensitive to it. We are at risk of always being 'on the look-out' for it. It is not difficult to see how this can apply to pain.

What if we took the same approach to chronic pain? Instead of trying to avoid it or escape from it, what if we deliberately faced it for an extended period? This would mean accepting the presence of pain without trying to minimise it with medication.

We have been trying this method with our patients for many years. After a while, those who practise it a lot find the pain doesn't bother them as much. Of course, it's not easy for everyone and some say they can't face even the idea of doing it. In those cases one-to-one sessions with a psychologist may be needed to master it. But overall, we have found this method very helpful in lessening the distress caused by pain. The pain will remain but you can train yourself to be less bothered by it.

We recommend you practice focussing on the pain in this way whenever your pain starts to trouble you. A good time to practice is when you are exercising or doing other activities that can aggravate your pain. Try it when you are trying to go to sleep and feel you can't get comfortable.

To begin with, you might like to combine it with your relaxation practice. Start with a mix of long and short sessions. We recommend two or three twenty minute sessions a day. In between, you should try brief sessions (1–2 minutes) whenever you notice your pain through the day, as when you are exercising. After a few weeks it will become a habit and you will find yourself doing it without realising it.

Start by letting go and calming yourself with your relaxation technique, but focus your attention on your pain. Focus on your pain as calmly as possible. Make no effort – just allow yourself to feel the pain sensations without reacting to them. You can even imagine you are immersing yourself in the pain, like getting into the water at the beach or pool – remember how it often seems hard to start with but after a few minutes our body adjusts. Desensitising is a similar process, but you are learning to adjust to an internal sensation.

Most importantly, you don't need to think. Just observe the sensations for what they are – sensations with no real meaning and they are not harming you. Try not to block the pain or even think about how bad it is. You can't stop yourself thinking but you don't have to respond to the thoughts. Just let any thoughts pass you by. It is especially important to avoid cursing the pain – that risks giving it a special status and extra power. Just calmly focus on that sensation you call pain and see what happens.

You can keep reminding yourself that you are OK and the pain doesn't mean anything, just harmless signals in your nerves.

Try to keep your attention on the pain. Don't try to change the pain or even try to make it go away – as that is still trying to escape from it. Calmly, let it be there and continue relaxing.

Initially, the pain may start to feel more severe. This just because you're used to trying to get away from it, but this effect will pass. Try not to let it stop you. Remind yourself that it can't cause you any damage. You are OK. Keep going because it won't continue getting worse. Any increase in pain will settle (after all you are not doing anything that can harm you).

After each session spend a minute or so thinking about what you noticed. Try not to measure it in terms of 'did it work' or 'did it make the pain go away', rather what did you notice? Compare that with the last time you did it. Over time you should start to notice changes in the way you experience your pain at these times. You might like to experiment with the technique.

It can help you to get into regular practice by keep a record of how much your pain bothers you before and after each session. Make a copy of the recording form like this one below:

As you get better at the technique try using it to counteract your pain whenever you find it starting to intrude.

One word of caution. We don't recommend that you use the technique to over-ride your normal pacing of activities. You should continue to pace activities that aggravate your pain, but use the desensitising technique to cope with your pain whenever it starts to trouble you.

Pain Desensitisation Record Sheet

Please rate how much the pain bothers you
before and after each long session (3/day).

Rate **how much it bothers you** from 0–10,
where 0 = 'does not bother me at all' and
10 = 'extremely distressing').
Place a tick (✓) in the last box for all brief sessions.

Day	Distress 0-10)		Distress (0-10)		Distress (0-10)		Brief sessions
	Start	End	Start	End	Start	End	(√)

Overall, it is best to approach these techniques as realistically as possible – don't expect too much too soon – but do try each of them as often as possible. After a while you will find one or two will be quite helpful at times, providing you remember to go on using them. Including these techniques in your relaxation practice is often a good way to start, but relaxing first isn't essential. You'll find that as you get better at desensitizing you also become more relaxed when feeling your pain.

Improving Sleep
14

Sleep problems are often reported by people with chronic pain. It can be trouble getting to sleep or staying asleep (or both). Many report broken sleep, where they wake up every hour or two through the night. Others say they often wake up early in the morning and can't get back to sleep.

Some say, they just can't get to sleep until very late at night and then they sleep in late the next morning. Others find they almost become nocturnal, being unable to sleep at night but dozing off during the day.

Many blame these sleep problems on their pain ("the pain wakes me when I roll over"), or they have trouble getting comfortable. Others say that troubling thoughts interfere with getting to sleep. In these cases, they may be worrying about financial matters or worrying about not getting a decent sleep again.

Effects of lack of sleep
Ongoing poor sleep can leave us feeling quite run down and generally tired or 'out of sorts' for much of the time. We can become more irritable and our pain more of a burden. We all know how much easier it is to deal with day to day hassles and pain when we have had a good night's sleep. Many people with chronic pain end up sleeping whenever they can, even in the middle of the day. This can compound the problems of chronic pain leading to more social withdrawal and worse night time sleep.

Poor sleep can lead to worse sleep, especially if we start to worry whether or not we will get to sleep each night. That can become a self-fulfilling prophesy (making it even more likely that there will be a problem).

What to do about it

You may have tried all sorts of remedies, such as drinking hot milk at night, avoiding coffee, counting sheep or listening to relaxation tapes. None may seem to make any real difference. If you have seen your doctor about it, you may have been given some medication to see if that might help. You might have tried many different types of medication. Some may seem to work for a while, but then wear off. Sometimes, when you have the odd good night it can be difficult to work out why it happened. It may have been just luck. Before we look at your options, let's quickly think about normal sleep.

Normal sleep

Many people say they need 8 hours a night, but normal sleep patterns change with age. Typically, the main changes occur from around 20 to 60 years of age when they tend to stabilise, especially in healthy people. Older adults usually go to bed earlier and wake earlier than younger adults. They also have more trouble adjusting to time changes like shift work and jet-lag. Older people also tend to be more easily disturbed while sleeping.

Normal sleep has different stages, from light to deeper sleep (when it is harder to be awoken). Each stage lasts about 90 minutes and the deepest stage is usually in the first half of the night. We can also have periods of wakefulness which vary in length and frequency, but they often increase with age. So, it is normal to sleep deeply at times and have periods of being slightly awake as well. We need to recognise this and not see it as a problem. If we over-react to the wakeful periods we risk undermining the quality of our sleep. Let's consider the options for improving the quality of our sleep.

(1) Medication

Drugs for sleep should only be used after consulting your doctor. It is very important that you don't use drugs prescribed for some-one else. The most obvious reason for this is that the drugs may be dangerous for you to take. It is also quite possible that someone else's drugs are not the best way for you to deal with your sleep problems. Discussing the issues with your doctor will help you to make an informed decision. It may well be the case that med-ication is not the only or best way for you to deal with your sleep problems.

There are two main groups of medications that are often used to help with sleep.

(i) The tricyclic anti-depressants

These come under a number of brand names. These drugs are normally used to help improve mood. But one of their side effects is drowsiness. This means that if this medicine is taken at night it can help us to get to sleep. This can be achieved with smaller doses than those normally used for when people feel depressed. Like all medication, before you decide to take them it is impor-tant to be aware of any possible side effects and precautions. In the case of tri-cyclic antidepressants many find that they feel "hungover" or have difficulty "getting going" the next day. Other side effects are blood pressure falling, dry mouth and difficulty passing water.

(ii) Benzodiazepines

These are a group of drugs which include diazepam(Valium), temazepam(Temaze) and lorazepam(Ativan). While they can help you to get some sleep, they should be used carefully and usually for no longer than about one week. They are habit-forming and it can be difficult to stop taking them. They can become less effective after a few weeks or they can make your sleeping pattern even more disturbed. In fact, the sleep you get may not be as restful as normal sleep and many people report waking up the next morning feeling groggy or hungover. However, you could argue that some is better than none. That may be true for a short period, but it is not recommended as a long-term option. It is usually better to look at possible reasons for your poor sleep and other options for dealing with them.

Another problem with these drugs is that they can stay in your body for a couple of days and cause side effects, such as affecting the way you think. Clearly not a good idea! If you are trying to learn the approaches in this book we strongly advise that you take these drugs only for a short period of time and work closely with your doctor on limiting their use.

Other drugs and alcohol

It shouldn't need to be said, but using alcohol (with or without the other drugs mentioned here) as a means of improving sleep is to be strongly discouraged. It is not helpful and risks potentially dangerous interactions with other drugs. The resulting sleep is seldom restful and usually leaves you feeling 'hungover' the next morning.

Some other drugs for pain do contain a calmative agent (eg. Syndol), and may be used to help sleep. Caution is recommended in these cases as you are really taking three other drugs (Codeine, caffeine and Paracetamol) that you may not need, especially on a long-term basis.

(2) Other options – does anything work?

To answer this question a good place to start is to keep a record of your current sleep patterns. If you do this for a week or so, it can help you to see where you are having trouble and whether or not there is any pattern to it. Sometimes, we may be surprised to learn that we actually are sleeping more than we thought. The problem in these cases may be more one of the quality of the sleep, how refreshing it was, for example. Some people report than even a long medication-induced sleep can leave them feeling quite hung-over the next morning.

Whereas others seem to find a short cat-nap gives them a bit of a lift.

Copy this sleep chart onto a piece of paper or into a diary and monitor your sleep pattern for a week or so.

SLEEP CHART

Day/Date	Lights out time	Wake up time	No. of times awake	How rested? (0–10 rating)	Comments
				Rate from 0–10 where 0 = not rested and 10 = fully rested	anything relevant
Example: Monday, April 10	10.45pm	6.30am	3	4	couldn't get comfortable, too much noise outside

Keep track of your sleep by filling it in each morning. It is usually best to keep it beside your bed, so you will fill it in soon after waking.

After recording your sleep pattern for a few days you should have a clearer idea of where the problems lie. It might be repeated waking through the night, or having trouble getting to sleep. This observation should help you to work out the best way to deal with the problem. A list of common reasons for poor sleep and recommended good sleep habits is set out below, but before you try ways of improving your sleep it is important to realise there are no "quick fixes" for sleep problems. Most attempts to improve long-term sleep problems will take up to several weeks of <u>consistent</u> application of the strategies before improvements may be seen. It can help to remember that your sleep may well have taken some time to get to where it is now, expecting to overcome the effects of this quickly is generally unrealistic. More likely, it will be a process of trial and error until you find what suits you best.

Common Causes of poor sleep	Options
Daytime naps	Avoid them, restrict sleep to evenings
Too much resting during the day	Try to keep generally active, physically and mentally, through the day
Worries, stress	Deal with worries before bed, or write them down and decide to address them tomorrow. Use your relaxationtechnique and mental distractions. If you can't sleep after 20–30 minutes get up and do something peaceful until feeling ready for sleep again, then return to bed
Medication (misuse or withdrawal)	If you stop your pain killers or tranquilisers, it can take a few days to a week or so before they are out of your system. So remind yourself that these effects will pass and that you are OK.
Stimulants before bed (coffee, tea)	If these are a problem, stop taking them in the evenings (replace them with warm drinks which don't contain caffeine).
Pain, discomfort	If you have paced your activities during the day your pain will not usually be as bad as when you overdo things, so you could prevent some of the pain. Often pain seems to feel worse at night anyway, partly due to there being no distractions for us to focus on. In this case, using relaxation and desensitizing can help. Dealing with any distressing thoughts with thought challenging is also important.

Common Causes of poor sleep	Options
Alcohol or large meals in the evening	Avoid or limit the amount and only drink with dinner Reduce the amount of food eaten at night.
Depression, anxiety	Long-standing depression will take a while to resolve, but thought challenging is helpful and may be supplemented by antidepressant medication. Anxiety can be addressed by using relaxation, desensitization, and thought challenging. You can use the strategies outlined in this book (or the others we have recommended) to deal with both depression and anxiety.
Trying too hard to sleep (lying in bed tossing and turning, getting frustrated)	Use your relaxation technique, but if it's not working get up and do something relaxing or peaceful until ready to return to bed. You may need to repeat these several times, but try to stay as calm as possible. Remember, if you are relaxing you are still getting rest.
Engaging in activities late at night which get your brain going too fast (e.g. preparing your income tax return)	Try to plan to avoid these types of tasks at night if at all possible. Plan to do more relaxing, pleasant tasks last in the day (reading, listening to music, etc.).
Going to bed at irregular hours or often sleeping in late in the mornings	Try to establish a regular routine at night (eg. getting ready to go to bed about the same time each night, first clean your teeth, then have a glass of water, then get undressed for bed and avoid watching TV or reading in bed). Try to get up at about the same time each day, regardless of how you feel.
Bedroom too warm/cold; or used for too many non-sleep activities.	Adjust temperature to slightly cool; use bedroom mainly for sleep and sex – not as an office

Good sleeping habits

In addition to the points listed above, there are a number of basic guidelines for getting enough sleep. These points are not going to be equally helpful for everyone, but amongst this list you should find something that could help.

1. Establish a regular routine before retiring for the night.
This can help you prepare for sleep. Try to go to bed around the same time each night. For example, put the cat out, turn out the lights through the house, clean your teeth, undress for bed, get into bed and do your last relaxation or desensitization session for the day.

2. If you are often kept awake by worry, try these steps:
- The first rule is that telling yourself to stop worrying is usually unsuccessful. Instead, it usually helps to do something else.
- Get a pen and some paper. Write down the worries or problems that are on your mind
- Then write down the next step you think you could take towards sorting out the problem and leave it until the morning.
- If you wake up during the night worrying about the problem, remind yourself that you have the matter in hand, and that going over it now will not help. If a new worry crops up in the night, write it down and deal with it the next day.
- Practice your relaxation and desensitization techniques. If you prefer you could also and try to focus your mind on a distracting image or scene (eg. remembering a previous holiday or imagining somewhere that you would like to go).
- If these steps are not helping within 20–30 minutes, it may be better to get up for a while and do something relaxing (so avoid stimulating activities like computer games, Crosswords, or an exciting TV program). Options include reading, listening to music, practising your relaxation technique. When you are ready, return to bed and see what happens (remember, don't try to sleep). After a while, if you still find yourself lying there feeling restless, get up again and repeat the same types of activities.
- If possible, make sure the room temperature is cooler rather than hotter.

3. Make your bed and bedroom as associated with sleep as possible

- try not to use your bedroom during the day, except for relaxing.
- go to bed or turn the lights out only when you are sleepy and within a limited time period, such as 9 pm to midnight.
- if possible, make sure the room temperature is cooler rather than hotter.
- If after 20 minutes or so you haven't fallen asleep, it could be worth getting up and leaving the bedroom for a while (see section above).
- Apart from sleeping and sex, try to avoid doing other things in bed, like watching TV, phone calls or writing letters.

4. Try not to "clock watch"
This will only make things worse. Turn your clock's face away from you.

5. If you are coming off some tablets
Check if this could cause temporary sleep problems. This information could help you to prepare for such problems and to reassure you that they will settle as your body is cleared of the tablets. With some tablets (especially tranquillisers), this may take time.

6. Establish a regular routine for the mornings.
To help your 'biological clock' get into a regular pattern it can help to try to get up at the same time each day, even when you don't feel like it.

7. When you do have a difficult night (and they will happen)
Try to put some thought into why it might have happened. Rather than jump to conclusions (such as, "Oh, it's no good, see I do need my tablets"), it could well be that the poor night was due to the withdrawal effects of the sleeping tablets or perhaps you over-looked some of the points mentioned above. Sometimes, of course, it will just be one of those nights that happens to all of us. Whatever

the case may be, by not over-reacting you will be less worried about it the next night, which will help to make that night more successful. Remember, like relaxation, you can't force yourself to sleep, but we can do a great deal to improve it.

8. Keep a record of your progress each night (using the sleep chart).

This can help to remind you that overall your sleep is improving, even if it doesn't always feel like it. After a week or two you can look back and you will usually see that things are gradually getting better, while the problem nights are getting fewer. If this is not happening then try to work out why. If you feel unsure how to proceed, perhaps you could discuss it with your doctor or psychologist.

REMEMBER,
It will take time for these methods to help you improve your sleep.

It is vital, therefore, that you stick to these methods for some time, even if progress is slow.

Stress and Problem Solving

What is stress?

S tress is one of those things that is hard to define, although we can recognise it in ourselves.

Stress can be thought of as **the way we feel**. For example, when we feel very tense or worried, or when we feel we are working under pressure.

Stress can also be reflected in the **way we behave**, such as when we are irritable, having trouble concentrating or smoking/drinking a lot more than usual.

Stress can also be linked to the **pressures in our internal and external environment**. So, **pain is a source of stress**, just like having too many bills to pay or too much to do in too short a time.

Sometimes people say that **things are stressful when they feel they don't have any control over them**. For example, being late for appointments because the trains don't arrive on time. Lack of a sense of control is one of the things that people troubled by persisting pain often report as one of the stressful aspects about their pain.

While stress is often seen as bad, it can be useful too.
For example, many of us feel that we perform better under some pressure, rather than no pressure at all – even if we don't want to admit it. Think about when you would have got something done if

there was no time limit. Common examples are things like tidying the house when friends are coming to dinner, or students completing assignments only when the deadline is coming up. Governments are the same – how many useful community projects suddenly get done just before an election?

Similarly, lying on a deserted beach in the tropics will usually be appealing to someone running from the rain on a cold winter's day in a big city. But, if you lie on that beach too long, you might be nice and relaxed, but apart from being sunburnt you could also find that your muscles have become weaker and your joints stiffer. If we don't make our muscles and joints do some work every day, after a while they will tend to lose condition and become weak and stiff.

Some stress (or pressure on us to do things) actually helps us to stay alive and our bodies (and minds) to function properly.

Stress can also be a problem
However, stress can be a problem if we have too much of it. This often happens when we feel the pressure on us is more than we can manage. These are the times when we can get irritable or feel overwhelmed.

The aim of stress management
The aim of stress management is therefore not to eliminate stress, but rather to help you feel you can manage despite all the pressures on you.

Why do we feel stressed?
The amount of stress you feel is likely to be influenced by three types of things:

1. The stressful situation
In general, the bigger, the more unexpected, the more unfamiliar the stressful situation, the more stressful it will be. For example, having your socks stolen is likely to be less stressful than

discovering your house has been burgled. Also, knowing in advance that your train will be delayed is likely to be less stressful than when it happens unexpectedly.

With regards to persisting pain,
would it be more or less stressful if you didn't know why you have pain?

Would it be more or less stressful if you thought it was due to something life-threatening?

Would it be more or less stressful if you thought it meant you could end up in a wheel chair?

2. How you see the problem and your ability to cope
If you see the problem as unimportant, then you are unlikely to feel stressed by it. But if you see it as very important to you then you are more likely to feel stressed or troubled by it. However, if you feel you know how to deal with the problem, then you are less likely to be stressed by it than if you feel you won't be able to cope.

With regards to persisting pain,
would it be more or less stressful if you thought it wouldn't interfere with your work or lifestyle?

Would it be more or less stressful if you thought you could cope with it, no matter how bad it got?

3. The level of helpful support available from friends/relatives
If you feel you have helpful and understanding friends or relatives around, you are less likely to feel stressed by a problem than if you feel alone and without support.

With regards to persisting pain,
would it be more or less stressful if you had no one for support?

On the other hand, how would you feel if your family took over everything for you and left you feeling completely useless?

Just having family or friends around doesn't automatically mean they will be helpful. At times, they can add to the burden. The chapter on relationships discusses some of these issues.

Overall,

The amount of stress you feel doesn't just depend on what has happened to you. For example, if you have a supportive relationship with your family or friends and your pet cat is run over on the road you are likely to suffer much less than a lonely pensioner who is living alone and whose only friend, a pet cat, is run over. You will both suffer to some extent, but you will probably suffer less than the lonely pensioner. The reasons for that are that the cat didn't mean as much to you as it did to the lonely pensioner and you have friends and family around to provide comfort for you – the lonely pensioner may not.

How to manage stress

Using the three points mentioned above you can improve the way you manage (or cope with) stresses in your life. Remember, the aim of stress management is to find ways of dealing with stresses so that they are manageable and not overwhelming. It is unlikely, as well as undesirable, that we can or should get rid of stress completely.

1. Deal with the causes of the stress

If possible, it could help to deal with the cause of the stress. For example, if you find that you are becoming irritated by the volume of your neighbour's TV, asking them to turn it down would probably solve the problem. Similarly, if you are becoming concerned that the brakes on your car are not working properly, getting them checked by a mechanic should help to sort things out.

However, it is often not possible to deal effectively with the cause of the stress. For example, if you have a car accident you can't do much about it – it has happened and can't be undone.

Chronic pain is another common cause of stress which often cannot be removed completely.

2. Change the way you are looking at the problem

When you can't remove the cause of the stress you might be able to change with the way you are looking at it or the way you are reacting to it.

(a) Look at what you are saying to yourself

Sometimes you might realise you are viewing the cause of the stress too negatively. In which case it could help to stop for a moment and think of an alternative, more helpful way of looking at the problem.

For example, if you are running late for an appointment you might find yourself feeling upset and worrying that the person you were going to see would think you were thoughtless or unreliable. Such thoughts are likely to make you feel even more upset. What's more they may not be accurate and they won't make you get there faster – unless you become completely unconcerned about whether you get there or not (in that case, the other person would have grounds for thinking you were unreliable).

If you could challenge these thoughts (look at how accurate or how helpful they were) and then try to view the situation in other, more helpful, ways it might help to lower your level of distress. In this example, you could challenge these thoughts by saying (to yourself) things like:
- "He might think I'm thoughtless and unreliable, but it's unlikely because I'm normally on time, and I always turn up or ring to say I can't make it".
- "Even if he does think I'm thoughtless or unreliable, it would be inaccurate and he should understand when I explain the reason for my lateness".

- "If he doesn't understand or won't listen to my apologies-
  it doesn't mean his view of me is right (perhaps he is
  over-stressed)".

Whenever you are feeling stressed it is worth taking a few
moments to stop and consider how you are viewing the problem.

> **Are your thoughts inaccurate?**
> **Are they unhelpful?**
> **Are they too negative?**
> **Are they too positive?**

If your answer to any of these questions is **Yes** then challenge
them, think of another way of viewing the problem. In particular,
think of a way of viewing the problem which is more helpful.

**The point of this is that if you get a clear idea of what the
problem is then you are more likely to be able to deal with it
effectively.** If you see a problem in too negative a way you could
be making things harder than they need to be. But equally, if you
see it as too positive (too rosy) you might just be "pulling the wool
over your own eyes" (that is, deceiving yourself) and as a result,
you may not deal with the problem as effectively as you might. This
could lead to more problems later.

(b) Look at how you are trying to cope
   Are you using your **relaxation technique**? Stop for a moment
   and spend a minute or two relaxing until you feel a bit calmer
   and more in control of yourself. The clarity of your thinking
   will probably improve too.

   Are you trying to do too much in too short a time? If so,
   stop and spend a few moments putting things in order of priority. Do what is most important first, then the next most
   important and so on.

Are you getting stressed by the same (or similar) things repeatedly? If so, take some time out to think about how you are dealing with them. Perhaps, it's the way you are going about it. What changes could you make? For example, sometimes you might find that you are repeatedly getting stressed because you put things off until the last minute and then run out of time. In this case you could try to prevent the problem recurring by planning to do things sooner rather than later, or spreading it out over a longer time rather than waiting until the last minute.

3. Enlist the help of family or friends

If you already have helpful family or friends then that is fortunate and should prove of great benefit for you at times of stress. Remember, though, they will find it easier to help if you **tell them clearly what the problem is and how you would like them to help**. [Expecting people who are close to us to read our minds when we have a problem is often the cause of mis-understandings.]

If your family or friends are not very helpful at times of stress then it may be worth your while (and their's) if you tried to look at why this was the case. When things are calmer, it could be worth sitting down with them to discuss your concerns and how you see things at these stressful times. It may be that they see these situations differently to you, and neither of you have realised that. That doesn't necessarily mean that one is right and one is wrong, just that you have seen things differently. Perhaps you might now be able to reach some agreement on these situations and how you could handle them better.

In the long-run, putting time and effort into improving and maintaining our close relationships will also help, but won't, of course, guarrantee a trouble-free life.

Usually improvements in our relationships can only be achieved through the joint efforts of both parties. However, this can be helped by reading a suitable book on assertiveness or communication skills [see the end of this chapter for some useful books on these topics]. In some cases, it can be worthwhile to seek some professional assistance through a suitable counsellor – who would have the advantage of being more objective about the problems in your relationship [in Australia, Relationships Australia have offices throughout the country and are a good place to start looking for professional help for relatively little cost].

Alternatively, if you feel that the chances of being able to improve your existing relationships are low then you could try to build new relationships. There are many ways of going about it. Sometimes you might just be lucky and run into someone at a pub or club, strike up a conversation and, over time, gradually become friends. A more reliable method could be to join a club or organisation connected with one of your interests. In this way at least you would be fairly confident of meeting people with whom you have something in common. Working with others is also a common means of building friendships.

It is important to remember that making and developing friendships is also a skill and needs thought and practice.

In conclusion

Stress or pressure on us to do things is a normal part of life. It is useful if it helps us to keep active and enjoying life. However, it can be a problem if we feel overwhelmed and unable to cope. When someone has chronic pain the normal stresses of daily life can make it even harder to deal with the problems caused by the chronic pain. It is therefore sensible to consider the ways in which you are dealing with the other stresses in your life. While you are probably managing most of these other stresses fairly well, it is possible that you could still make some improvements.

Re-read the points made in this section and see how you can apply them to the stresses in your life.

Problem solving

An important part of Stress Management is Problem Solving. This section provides practical guidance on a general approach to helping people deal with problems, whether they are related to pain or just the normal stresses and strains of daily life. The aims of this approach are:

1. To give you a method for tackling most problems.
2. To teach you a systematic method of dealing with problems, and
3. To improve your sense of confidence that you can cope.

When is problem solving applicable? **ANYWHERE. ANYTIME.** Whenever and wherever you have a conflict or demand on you to sort something out. The potential uses of problem solving are wide ranging, and include crisis-management, organisation of daily life, reducing distress and increasing effectiveness.

Naturally, dealing effectively with troubling pain also requires well-developed problem solving skills. In fact, it is our experience that those people who have these skills usually have much less trouble in managing their persisting pain.

If you follow the steps outlined below, you will be more likely to deal with difficult situations, including pain, in a constructive manner. As with all the skills outlined in this book, you will need to adjust them to your own circumstances, but that is a skill which requires practice too.

Steps involved in problem solving

1. Try to accurately describe the problem
Exactly what is it you are not happy with?
    Where and when is it occurring?
        What is involved?
            How often is it happening?

Clarifying the problem is the first step towards finding a solution.

For example, if you have been pacing up most of your activities through the day, but by the evening your pain is getting worse. You could say to yourself things like, "well I've been doing my pacing but it didn't work – my pain is worse than ever" "what's the point of doing all this?" "Maybe I should just give up."

These statements suggest you feel you've been doing everything as recommended, but not getting the results you expected. As a result you are feeling frustrated, disappointed and hopeless.

But is this the only way to look at what's happened? Is giving up your only or your best option?

Perhaps another way to look at this situation is to look at what you've been doing through the day. You might have been pacing most activities, but is the total amount of activity more than you usually do? If it is, then maybe you have really done too much today and that is why your pain is worse. If that's the case then you might be able to work out another solution besides giving up.

On the other hand, it could be that for some unknown reason your pain is just worse today. This can happen no matter what you do. So, it may not be your fault or the fault of the pacing method. In fact, if you had not paced, you might have been in more pain now.

Is it really accurate to say that your pain "is worse than ever"? But even if it is, does it really mean that there's no point in trying to achieve your goals? And does it mean you should give up? What could you do instead? What would you do if you "gave up"? Would that be any better?

Perhaps a more accurate assessment of things would be to say something like, "well my pain is worse tonight than usual. Maybe I've overdone things today. On the other hand, it could be just one of those days when my pain flares up for no good reason. This has happened lots of times before. I know it will settle soon, perhaps even by tomorrow."

2. Generate as many alternative options as possible.

What can you do about it? Try to come up with as many options as possible, regardless of how unlikely they may seem at first. It's a bit like having a menu to select from at a restaurant.

In the example given above, you could think back over the day and see if you really had over-done things. If that's the likely cause of your increased pain, at least you can work out how to avoid it happening again.

A good example of this was provided by one of our patients (we'll call him George) who really wanted to take his boat out to do some fishing. George hadn't been able to do this for a couple of years because of his back pain. After attending our programme he tried it again. Unfortunately, when he returned home from fishing the first time his pain was much worse. His wife said it looked like he would have to sell his boat. But George thought about why his pain had been stirred up and worked out that it could have been due to his sitting down while the boat bumped across the waves. As a result, he thought he might have been absorbing all the bumps through his body, especially his back, and that was why his pain was worse. A few days later George went out in the boat again. But this time instead of sitting down all the time, he stood up most of the time, and absorbed the bumps through his legs. This time when he got home his pain was no worse than usual and much better then it had been after the first trip. And he had managed to go fishing!

George could have said after the first attempt at going fishing that it was no use, his pain was worse, that doing our pain management programme hadn't helped. Instead, he used problem solving to think his way around a problem so he could achieve his goal of going fishing again.

In this example, some of George's options were:

1. Give up and sell the boat
2. Take more pain killers and still try to go fishing
3. Stand up when travelling in the boat rather than sitting down
4. Leave it a few weeks or months and try again
5. Wait for a calm day

George looked at each of these options and weighed up the pro's and con's of each. Then he tried option 3 and it worked.

3. Evaluate the alternatives.

Once you have made up your list of options for dealing with the problem you should then assess them – their advantages and disadvantages. Until you find one which seems the best. It may not be perfect, but it may be the best option available at present.

Try to be objective and realistic. Try taking into account both long and short term consequences.

In the example of George going fishing, if he had given up going fishing and sold his boat it would have meant giving up on his favorite leisure activity and he would have felt quite depressed at the loss. On the other hand if he had taken more pain killers and just gone fishing regardless, he would have had more pain after the trip, when the drugs had worn off and he would have ended up taking even more, which he wanted to avoid. Also, he was concerned about being out at sea full of strong pain killers. If they'd run into trouble he couldn't be sure that he would have managed. The other options of waiting, would only have meant putting it off without any guarantee that things would be any better in a few weeks or that a calm day would stay calm. In the end George felt that trying to go fishing but doing it differently offered him the best option and he was right.

4. Choose the best alternative.

What is the most appropriate, reasonable and practical option for you to take, in your present circumstances?

5. Make a plan

What are you aiming to do? How can you do it? What may make it difficult (and how could you get around these difficulties)? What resources do you have to implement your plan? Do you need help? What do you think you will need, (eg., money, tools, skills)?

6. DO IT.

Put your plan into action (as best you can). Use relaxation and challenge unhelpful thoughts if you are anxious and remember to pace yourself.

7. Assess the outcome.

Did your plan of action work? Did it have the effect you wanted? If **yes**, then do you want to do it again? If **no**, could you try one of the other alternatives, or generate some more?

Remember, **many problems do not have perfect solutions**. In many instances you can only try to do your best. At the end of the day, it can be more useful to learn from your mistakes than not to try at all. Always think about what you could do differently next time. Give yourself credit for what you did well and for trying.

Interacting with Those Around You 16

Most people who develop persisting pain find that having to manage pain can affect their close relationships with family and friends. Relationships with others, such as people at work or people serving you in a shop, can also be affected when you are trying to live with persisting pain. At times, others may find you more irritable than normal, or more withdrawn or reserved. In many cases people with chronic pain find their close relationships are put under great strain, but some report that working with those close to them to find ways around the problems caused by the pain can actually improve the relationships. In these cases, it is like bringing those involved closer together in their battle against a common foe.

We have seen many of the ways people feel that pain has affected their relationships. A few examples may give you a glimpse of what some people go through.

> Sally was convinced that her marriage was over because she felt her husband did not understand her pain problem. She felt he demanded her support, but didn't give her any in return. She wanted to get her life in order and to manage life with pain on her own terms. She separated from her husband, but he continued to keep in touch. For a while she thought about seeking counselling but without her husband's involvement. However, as she learnt to manage her pain more effectively, she realised that her lack of acceptance of her pain had

contributed to their relationship difficulties. She also came to recognise how her approach to dealing with her pain had had an adverse effect on their relationship.

In particular, while Sally had always tried to stay as independent as possible, doing as much as she could around the house and in other daily activities, at times she reached her limit and really needed her husband's help. But when she thought about how she had asked for help, she realised that often it was as though she had been expecting her husband to be able to 'read her mind'. There has since been a reconciliation between Sally and her husband. By learning to express herself more directly and clearly the misunderstandings have become much less common, and they both report they now feel more supported by each other.

Mary appeared to be the hub of her family's existence. Her ex-husband, teenage children, ageing parents, and an invalid relative were all a part of her busy day. Mary also continued to maintain her work but found it very difficult to cope without medication. Medication gave her some pain relief, but she used this to overdo activities and so she repeatedly aggravated her pain. She had difficulty asking others in the family to do what she had always seen as 'her duties', and she felt that no one else could ever do them as well as she could. Nevertheless, she felt resentful that she had to do everything. Unfortunately, while she could see how this approach was self-defeating, she felt she could not change it.

Larry lived with his fiancee. As his pain persisted they started to argue more. The arguments usually concerned things like his lying around and often sleeping through the day, his high medication use, and his unwillingness to socialise with their friends. His irregular attendance at work was also an increasing problem. Larry was reluctant to stop medication use and expected his fiancee to do everything in the home. Eventually, Larry learnt to manage his pain more effectively. He reduced, then ceased his reliance on medication and started to feel more in control of his pain. Despite his improvement his fiancee had

had enough, and the relationship was broken off. But Larry stuck at it, and he also worked on improving his ability to discuss issues without getting into a rage. Gradually, their relationship was rekindled. The couple found they both needed to make adjustments and have more realistic goals if their relationship was to survive.

Fifteen-year-old Robyn was in a wheelchair due to a back injury incurred playing sport. She was taking excessive amounts of morphine. Her mother, a nurse, was very involved in seeking treatment for Robyn. Her father worked long hours and so didn't see much of her. He said that he felt shut out and unable to help his daughter, and this contributed to his spending more time at work. In part, he put this down to the way her pain was being managed. He felt his wife and their doctor had largely taken over as appointments were during the day when he was at work, and he had little or no role to play. By the time they attended our clinic the whole family said they felt quite stuck and unsure of where to go.

When Robyn attended our ADAPT program her father was involved in driving her, a half-hour journey or more each way for three weeks. She was able to tell her father about the program as they travelled. Their relationship improved as he learnt more and she was able to show she was managing the problem independently. Their relationship is now much closer.

Whether or not these examples are familiar to you, they show how pain can become a major source of stress in a relationship. Recognising this and trying to do something about it will help not only yourself but also your family and friends.

In this chapter we will examine a number of common issues, including typical changes in relationships because of chronic pain, types of unhelpful communication, effective (assertive) communication styles, resolving conflict, the spouse or partner relationship, as well as parent–child relationship issues, and sexuality. In some situations it can be helpful to talk to a psychologist, social worker or counsellor about these issues.

When pain can be a problem in relationships

As your pain persists, anger, frustration and withdrawal may become a common feature of your behaviour towards those who love you. You may find you are unable to speak confidently or in a civil way at home or in social settings. You may have trouble saying no to invitations or requests, resulting in your feeling both resentment of others and a sense that you could be letting them down if you are unable to keep commitments. Others may feel rejected and unsure of you because of your behaviour and start avoiding you. With each failed interaction with the people around you the difficulties can increase. Your relationships may start to fall apart.

What are your options?

1 Ignore the problems and hope they will just go away—but what if they don't?
2 Leave—that might solve some of these problems in the short-term but what about your family? Is this really how you'd like to live?
3 Sit down with your family or someone you can confide in and try to work out why you are getting into these situations and the possible ways out of them.

If you took option 3, where might you start?

Goal setting

Before you make plans about changing your behaviour or other aspects of your daily life, it helps to work out where you want to end up—your goals. Dealing with relationship issues is no different. As you did in your original goal setting exercise, why not write down some of the goals that you would like to achieve in your close relationships?

As you do this, consider not just identifying problems but the way to actually say how you would like the improvements to look. It usually helps if you can describe your goals as specifically as possible, such as what you would like to do, when or in what situation. For example:

- 'I don't want to shout at the kids so much' may be better phrased as, 'I want to speak more calmly to the kids, especially when the pain is bad'.
- 'I really want Mum to stop giving me advice about what treatments to have for my pain' may be better phrased as, 'I want to tell Mum I have learnt how to manage my pain problem and I would like her to encourage me with my efforts'.
- 'I want to talk to my partner about our sex life' may be better phrased as 'I would like to tell my partner how much I care about him or her and talk about the best ways to have sex, now I know how to cope better with pain'.

Other common interactions with others which you might want to improve include those you have at work, at home, with friends and with children.

1 **At work.** You may no longer be working or you may be working reduced hours, or be on light duties. This may have had an effect on the attitude of your co-workers, reflecting their scepticism or bias against someone who doesn't 'pull their weight'. Your employer may be frustrated with your reduction in productivity and increasing absences. How could you deal with these situations? It is possible that you will never convince some people that you have chronic pain and, as a result, have limitations to what you can do. With those people this may be a battle that isn't worth fighting. On the other hand, there are many people, including employers, who can be responsive to hearing your side of the story and will be prepared to help or to make allowances for you if they are given an idea of what it would involve and for how long. So, working out ways of telling others about your pain and how you have learnt to manage it could be worthwhile.

2 **At home.** You may experience a loss of self-esteem as you are no longer fulfilling your role as breadwinner or equal contributor. Other changes may include reduction in your standard of living, and recreational and social interests. If your spouse or

partner was not working, he or she may be forced to return to work to make up for your lost income. Equally, if he or she was already working they may need to work longer hours to earn more for the family. At the same time, you may not be able to take over all of their old duties around the house because of your pain. The effect on you may be one of guilt, loss of confidence and self-esteem, anger and frustration. How might you address these issues with your spouse or partner in a constructive way?

3 **With friends.** Decreased socialising may occur because of financial constraints, physical inability to participate in social and recreational pursuits, unwillingness to commit to or 'stay the distance' when socialising due to pain. You may have lost interest in socialising with people. Yet, you might appreciate some consideration from your friends and you might want to maintain your links with them. How might you discuss these concerns with your friends?

4 **Children.** You may no longer be able to actively play with your children. Because of your mood the children may become unsure of your responses and so begin to avoid you in preference to dealing with your spouse. They may begin imitating your behaviour, reflecting anger, withdrawing and exhibiting pain behaviour. They may become protective of you. They may have fear because of hospitalisations and doctors 'doing things to you'.

Older children may become angry at doing your tasks and at your lack of involvement in their lives. Participation in family events such as cycling, picnics and holidays can suffer and the family may become accustomed to doing things without you. How could you deal with these concerns and re-establish your previously good relationships with your children?

Why might these problems be happening?

Before you try to come up with solutions to these problems, perhaps it would be worth your spending a little time working out why the problems are happening.

For example, is it likely they are all due to the others involved? While the problem could be caused by the other people, it is also possible that your responses are also contributing to the difficulties you are having with them. It is often difficult to be objective about ourselves (and our behaviour), but resolving interpersonal problems is usually helped by objective and honest assessment of ourselves.

Most interpersonal conflicts involve at least two people. It is likely that in your case your behaviour is at least part of the problem. That doesn't mean it will be all your fault, but rather, if you could change your approach in some way it might help the others involved to change as well. You may not be able to control the behaviour of other people but you should be able do something about your own.

Have a look at this list of behaviours you may engage in when other people are about. Regardless of how the behaviour started, do you ever do any of the things mentioned here when your pain is troubling you?

- *Withdrawing verbally*—not talking, not making conversation, ignoring others, not explaining what is happening, almost expecting others to read your mind, not indicating how they might help.
- *Withdrawing physically without explanation*—leaving the room, going to the bedroom, to the shed, or 'out'.
- *Exhibiting pain behaviours*—such as grimacing, holding, groaning, complaining about your pain.
- *Talking about your pain*—and how terrible it is.
- *Loss of interest in others*—not responding to others, lack of awareness of others and their concerns.
- *Mood changes*—irritability, anger, frustration, despondency, sadness.
- *Provocative statements*—such as 'You don't know how bad this is', 'I can't ... because I'm in pain', and 'If you had pain like this you would understand'.

Faced with such behaviour from you, others may feel unsure how to help. If you often behave in these ways with others despite their attempts to help, they may start to feel rejected by you and even helpless. Over time, they may start to withdraw from you.

Of course, from your point of view you may feel that as they don't have pain like yours they really don't understand. You may also feel that you have no choice, almost as if the pain is making you behave like that, or that if you didn't behave in these ways you might do or say something you'd regret. But are these responses your only option? Let's examine these views.

If they did have pain like yours, how much difference would it really make to how they behaved towards you? At our clinic we have seen many pain patients who did not get on with each other. Once they'd got to know each other, the fact that they all had pain didn't seem to make them more sympathetic to each other. A number of patients have even commented to our staff that they are getting fed up with the antics of some other patients.

It is possible, then, that the reason your family or friends are starting to withdraw from you is not that they don't understand what it is like to have pain, but rather they don't know how to help you. Especially if you won't tell them or discuss it with them. Like all of us, your family and friends can't read your mind. You too may not know how they could help, but it might be a start to at least tell them that. Then you might be able to start discussing your options with them.

It might help to know about some recent research on pain patients and their spouses, which has shown that good supportive relationships are often those where the person in pain is encouraged to do as much as they can manage but the spouse helps out on certain tasks, especially those that are usually difficult, like taking out the bin or vacuuming. In addition, the spouse in these relationships will often help when the spouse in pain specifically *asks* for assistance. This avoids the spouse in pain expecting their spouse to either read their mind or to just take over everything. Providing practical help when it is needed rather than taking over everything enables the spouse in pain to still feel useful. It also means their limitations are being acknowledged.

Relationships where conflict and tensions can run high are often those where either the spouse of the pain patient takes over everything, but resents it, or the spouse withdraws and does very little to help. So what options do you have when your pain is troubling you and you want to avoid the sorts of behaviours listed earlier, especially when the people around you are important to you?

- *Instead of withdrawing verbally,* try telling those you are with that your pain is troubling you and you don't mean to be rude but you might be quieter than usual for a period. Still, you do want to hear what is going on. You might even ask if they could help by sitting down to talk rather than standing up, as you find that difficult.
- *Instead of withdrawing physically* and without explanation, try explaining that your pain is troubling you. Ask them to excuse you for a short period while you go and do your stretch or relaxation exercises. Tell them you will be back shortly.
- *Instead of exhibiting pain behaviours,* try minimising such behaviours or building them into more 'non-pain' behaviours, such as changing position, getting up or stretching.
- *Instead of talking about your pain and how terrible it is,* try to avoid talking about your pain as much as possible. You may agree in advance with those close to you that you will let them know when it is bad and you need help with something, but apart from that you would prefer to be treated normally.
- *Instead of losing interest in others,* try making an effort to listen to what others are talking about and to ask them questions about themselves. After all, you may find it helps to get your attention off your pain.
- *Instead of accepting mood swings,* try using the methods outlined in this book. In particular, you could challenge any unhelpful thoughts you may be having, replacing them with more helpful alternatives. You could also be practising your relaxation technique and trying to calm yourself.

- *Instead of making provocative statements,* try checking such statements before they are out of your mouth, or apologising for them if they have already slipped past your guard. Challenging such thoughts before they are spoken could also help to modify such unhelpful views. Put yourself in the position of the other person in these situations—how would you respond to such statements? If you really feel that others don't understand, why don't you ask them about it? It may help to resolve an unnecessary problem you are having with them. For example, you might say something like 'When I say my pain is bad, I often get the feeling that you want to withdraw from me. Is that how you see it?' This sort of question doesn't accuse the other person of anything, so they shouldn't feel defensive and clam up. Rather, you are simply stating how you feel or how you see things and you would like to discuss it with them. Such a method often makes it possible to discuss even quite sensitive subjects without too much heat being generated.

These suggestions are only that—suggestions and not statements carved in stone. But they do show that there are many ways you can behave towards others when your pain is troubling you. The alternatives can avoid creating tensions and misunderstandings with those close to you.

Good communication with others is not, of course, confined to pain issues. Good or effective communication with others is important to the maintenance and development of all aspects of our relationships. If you have never really given much thought to how you communicate with others it might be useful to think about some basic aspects of good communication skills. You might also like to read more comprehensive books about the topic. Again, see your local library or bookshop for suitable books.

Basic principles for assertive communication

Assertive communication does not mean being aggressive. Instead, it means saying what you want to say in a way that is clear but respectful of others. Shouting orders at someone may be clear but it probably isn't respectful of others and it could alienate them from you. Equally, assertive communication doesn't mean manipulating other people to get what you want. You may have expressed yourself very clearly and you may have done it in a respectful way, but the other person may still disagree with you or not want to do what you have asked—that is their right.

Communication skills are learnt, we are not born with these skills. So if you feel you are not a good communicator you can still improve—with practice. Practice of these skills is essential. Simply reading about them and thinking they make sense is not enough for you to be able to use them. Try to practise these skills alone to begin with (like an actor rehearsing lines), and later with those you are close to (explaining what you are doing first and seeking feedback from them to help you improve). In general, good communication requires:

- *Knowing what you want to say*—that is, the main points you are trying to make
- *Getting your message across in a form that is understandable*—that is, clear, audible, and appropriate to the situation. This may be helped by making eye contact and using facial expression, such as a smile or frown
- *Listening to the other's responses* (to ensure they heard you correctly and you have heard their response clearly). It may help to repeat back to the other person what you thought they said, just to make sure you understood their response correctly

Of course, there is much more to good communication, depending on the situation. For example, one area many people have particular trouble with is trying to resolve a dispute with their spouse, partner or family member. In situations like these, some additional points can be helpful.

1 **Try to stick to the subject** and avoid being distracted by other issues, or dragging in other issues yourself. In most relationships there will always be some unfinished business from the past and you will never run out of things to drag into an

argument, but then you will probably take a lot longer to resolve the present one.

2   **Try to remain as calm as possible.** Getting heated or upset is likely to affect your reasoning. Use your relaxation technique. If you feel you are having trouble remaining calm then maybe you should consider asking for a short break and returning to it when you feel more composed.

3   **Watch your body language** while you are talking or listening. If you look away when the other person is talking it can look as if you aren't listening. Equally, banging the table with your fist may be your way of emphasising a point, but it can be frightening to the other person. Keeping a calm voice, looking the other person in the eyes at the right time and not getting too physically close are all useful ways to complement your words.

4   **Try to show that you respect the other person**—for example, if you treat him or her as unimportant, they are unlikely to pay much attention to you. If you are having an argument, staying courteous with them and showing you are trying to listen to their point of view will often prove much more helpful than disregarding or rubbishing their statements. You can show you are listening by checking with the other person that you have understood what they have said. For example, you could say something like, 'So it sounds as though you feel that I am not doing as much as you would like around the house. Is that what you are saying?' Remember, other people don't have to do what you want—unless you are giving an order, like a policeman—it is up to them to decide how they will respond.

5   **Take care how you phrase expressions of strong negative feelings** such as anger or irritation. At these times it is often easy to slip into blaming the other person for how you are feeling. For example, saying things like 'You make me really mad', as if they have caused that feeling in you. If you think about it for a moment it is easy to see that no one really has the power to make us feel what they want us to feel.

The truth is that we may feel angry or irritated when someone does or says something we don't like or don't agree with. They may or may not be doing it to make us feel like that, but it is always up to us how we react. If you recall the discussion in Chapter 11, our feelings are usually strongly influenced by our perceptions—the way we see things or think about them. So other people really don't 'make us' feel anything. We may get upset or angry when another person does or says something we don't like or don't agree with, but how we react is up to us. Try not to accuse the other person of anything, because that risks putting them on the defensive and they may then focus on being affronted by your accusation rather than dealing with your concerns.

Instead, it can be more productive to try this sort of approach:

- Clarify what you thought they said, to make sure you have understood them clearly. It is possible you misheard or that they didn't realise how what they said came across to you. For example, you might say 'When you say that, it sounds like . . . Is that what you meant to say?' This gives the other person a chance to correct your impression.
- Respond to them bearing in mind the five points mentioned above. In general, it is more effective in these situations to state clearly when *you feel* upset or angry, *what your perception* of their behaviour or words is, and *how that affects you* and *how you feel* as a consequence. The words in italics should act as a guide to how you can deal with these situations with other people. We would recommend that you run a few of these sorts of conversations through your mind before you try them out on other people. Even try saying it to yourself in front of the mirror.

6 **Suggest ways of resolving conflict** once you are more confident about expressing your concerns more productively.
7 **Be aware of the timing of dealing with conflict**—just because you want to talk about it doesn't mean it is necessarily going to be acceptable to the other person. The consequences of

attempting to deal with conflict may result in a resolution, further work to be done or no resolution. If the latter is the case, at least you will know you have done your best for the time being.

Possible solutions for different family members

It is not possible to outline the types of problems everyone may face, let alone the best solutions. However, we have found that many pain patients have gained a great deal from listening to how other people in pain have dealt with common problems. The following pages outline some of the problems and the solutions which our patients have reported.

Spouse/partner relationship and the sexual relationship

Your partner may have experienced a number of significant changes in his or her role as a result of your injury and loss of function. These changes might include having to take on increased responsibility with family and tasks at home or having to increase their paid work to compensate for your reduction in earning capacity. They may have had to adjust to reduced socialising and recreational pursuits. They may also be experiencing a sense of loneliness within the relationship as a result of your focus on pain.

Common signs of 'wear and tear' in a relationship in these situations include spending less time together, a sense of having lost sight of your goals, resentment at the increased load, jealousy of partner who is working and socialising, and withdrawal leading to reduced conversation, reduced hugs and touching. There may also be more arguments about responsibilities, children's discipline, finances, as well as doubts about one's attractiveness to the partner and even concerns about their fidelity.

At the same time the sexual side of your relationship may have become more of a problem, resulting in your feeling more distant from your spouse or partner. Common difficulties people in chronic pain have reported in this area include fear of causing pain or

increasing pain (on the part of either partner), avoidance at bed-
time or withdrawing from each other, reduced libido and frequency
of intercourse, or failure to get an erection/ reach climax. You may
find you are both talking less about your sexual needs, or even
when you do try to have sex there may be difficulties finding comfortable positions. You may also have found that the medications
you have been taking affect your mood and sexual interest. Of
course, trying to cope with pain all day can also leave you feeling
you have little energy for engaging in sex. Finally, trying to explain
these issues to your partner or spouse is often difficult and can
easily be misunderstood as a form of rejection.

Most sexual difficulties in relationships are not due to issues of
performance or technique. Most are actually due to relationship
issues. These often need to be worked on before a good sex life
can be resumed. For that reason we have included a discussion of
sexual difficulties in this section on relationship problems. Of
course, most people with chronic pain will say that relationship
problems can still occur even if you don't have a sexual partner or
you are not concerned about sexual issues. Thus, the issues raised
here should still be relevant to anyone with chronic pain who is in
a relationship, whether it be with friends or family.

Broadly, the following points can be helpful, at least as a base
for starting to address these sorts of problems.

1 **Try to include your spouse or partner** when you are trying
   to problem solve or plan something—don't expect them to
   read your mind. Solving a problem together can help to bring
   you closer to each other.
2 **Try not to talk about pain all the time**—if in pain or having
   a flare up tell those who matter but don't dwell on it.
3 **Check and challenge your thoughts** when you are feeling
   irritable or angry.
4 **Acknowledge your partner's support** and his or her feelings—no one likes feeling ignored or being taken for granted
   (even if that's not your intention).

5 **Be prepared for difficulties** that your spouse or partner may have in adjusting to the changes you are making in improving how you manage your pain (such as when you start taking back some of your old roles in the relationship and family). Try to discuss these issues with him or her.

6 **Encourage your partner to allow you to try things again,** even if it will take longer or not be done as well (initially) than if they continued to do them.

7 **Set goals**—recreational and social—to do things together and with others. By doing this together rather than all by yourself the relationship can benefit as it is a simple way of bringing you together again.

8 **Manage your pain** with the strategies outlined in this book and tell your partner what you are doing about it. Ask him or her if they would like to read the book and discuss it with you). Discuss ways in which they could help you to implement your strategies.

9 **Talk as openly as possible** about any developing sexual problems. Try to avoid any sense of blame. Rather, try to work out possible solutions or things you might try together. This can be awkward to start with, but it usually gets easier as you work on it. Some people find that using humour—learning to laugh again, especially at yourself —can be a good 'ice-breaker' and reduce tensions. However, we recognise that this is not always appropriate and many people find it difficult due to the sensitivities involved. So don't feel that you have to make jokes about it. In fact, some people use jokes to hide their real feelings. In this case continuing to make jokes without really addressing the problems or concerns seriously can end up with your feeling you are not getting anywhere.

10 **Take the initiative in planning time together,** having fun, having sex. Don't always wait for your spouse or partner to bring up the issues. If you start getting apprehensive before having sex (or during) try to use your relaxation technique and challenge any unhelpful thoughts you may have. Sometimes

using fantasy (including erotic ones) images in your mind can also help to distract your attention from pain and possible problems. It can help to make sex more fun if you try new positions and even see it as a type of experiment. This can help to make you less self-conscious. If it works, great; if not, well there's nothing really lost, it was still fun trying. Talk as openly as possible (probably no one is ever completely open about these issues) about what you like or don't like. Honest feedback can mean that you don't waste time (and possibly, avoid resentment) on things you don't really like. Books on sex may help, but we do suggest that you make this fun and not take it too seriously. Alternatives to intercourse (intercourse isn't the only way to have enjoyable sex)—oral sex, masturbation, aids, even just stroking each other in non-genital areas, can all add to the sense of fun, but shouldn't be forced on your spouse or partner.

11 **Pace yourselves** in building tolerance to touching, stroking, and intercourse itself. Rushing in with expectations unrealistically high, especially if you have had a long period without sex, can set you up for disappointment. This can be discouraging for the next time.

12 **Romance**—show that you care, give compliments, make uninterrupted time for each other, special dinners, arrange a weekend away or on your own at home, give flowers, start getting to know each other again. Remember how much time you gave each other early in your relationship (and how enjoyable that was).

Relationships are usually salvageable but it does require both parties to want to work on it. Sometimes one or other partner will feel that things have gone too far to turn back. It may well be that separation could be the healthiest option to take—for both of you. However, this can be a very big step and shouldn't be rushed into. Talking things over with a counsellor or psychologist (or really just someone who is independent and to whom you feel you can talk) is usually a good idea at these times.

Singles with pain

You may have found that your circle of friends has diminished as you no longer participate in things like sports, work or other groups. You may also have lost touch with friends because you have withdrawn from them or because they are confused about your pain. They may not know how to relate to you and so have stopped including you. Equally, you may feel that they might get bored hearing about your pain or you may stop making arrangements with others because you have trouble keeping commitments. As a result they may feel that you have lost interest in them.

In situations like these, which are surprisingly common, you might decide not to do anything and just accept that there's nothing you can do about it. In that case it is unlikely that these situations would change. On the other hand you might decide to find new friends, perhaps with people who would be more understanding of your problems or not expect you to be the way you used to be. That might be easier said than done, as you would still be faced with working out ways of seeing the new friends despite your pain and the same issues that were a problem in your previous relationships could surface again. Alternatively, you might decide to re-establish your old relationships.

Whichever way you decide to go it can help to think about how you could achieve your goals. Some of the key points to consider here could be:

1 **Try to use the assertive skills** referred to earlier to acknowledge your part in the difficulties experienced in the relationship. If you decide to re-establish your friendships this would obviously involve telling your friends that you want to renew the friendships. Rather than say you are totally fine as a means of avoiding placing attention on your pain, it is usually helpful to explain that you have a pain problem, but you now know how to manage it.
2 **Be direct** in letting friends or potential partners know what you enjoy and are capable of. Do it in a way that does not put

responsibility onto the other person to 'do something for you' or to work out what you want.

3 **Take the initiative** if you want to be more sociable. Decide to do things that will bring you into contact with others. Joining a course or group that shares one of your interests is often a good place to start.

4 **Initiate fun** and encourage others to join you, rather than others needing to 'look after' you. Make and keep commitments like dates or evenings out, even if you have to modify plans as you go along.

5 **Be prepared to explain your limitations** in terms of sexual activity in a matter of fact way, pointing out what you can do to still have fun. Although this can be daunting in a new relationship, most people find that taking the initiative and explaining your situation to your partner as the relationship develops is usually better than waiting for them to ask you about it. If you leave it up to the other person to ask you why you are behaving in certain ways it is possible that they might be misinterpreting your behaviour. You can be honest without going into a lot of detail. Mostly, other people will want reassurance that you are okay and that they are not causing you any harm.

Of course, you may have to accept that you cannot win them all. Not all our relationships work out as we may wish. By taking the sorts of approaches outlined here at least you will have given yourself a good chance of establishing or re-establishing a relationship. If it doesn't work out you will probably have learnt something from it. However, if it's not working despite your best efforts it may well be better to conserve your energy for those who are interested in you (and whom you like as well).

Something for the spouse or partner of someone with chronic pain

As described in the previous chapter, it is quite likely that you also have been affected by your partner's pain problem and all that goes with it. You may have begun to feel resentful for the extra load at home and, possibly, increased care of children or other duties. You may have had to work longer hours or take on more work to help make up financial loss if your spouse or partner is no longer working. Reduced income can affect your quality of life and can become a cause of tension and arguments.

Your social life may have been eroded because your partner is unwilling or unable to commit to arrangements made. You have less time to 'do your own thing'. You may feel that no one ever seems to care about how you are, only about your partner. You may have trouble understanding what is actually wrong with your partner, his or her moodiness and depression, and why no one has been able to fix him or her.

You may feel that your partner is always talking about pain, or needing to be taken to doctors' appointments, treatment sessions and it may seem never-ending. You may begin to feel that your partner is 'out of it' mentally because of medication, and you may start to become concerned about the amount he or she is taking.

Your spouse or partner may start to withdraw from activities at home and shut themselves away in the bedroom. Conversations at home may become very limited.

You may start to feel quite resentful and even angry about your partner's ongoing condition. Over time, you might start to withdraw from him or her. You may also start to feel as though you can't talk about your own needs or how you are feeling or coping.

You may feel that you have to bear the brunt of your spouse's or partner's anger regarding pain, loss of work, loss of self-esteem, and so on. You might also start to feel that it is almost as though you can't have a normal lifestyle with your partner or spouse.

In situations like these your options may appear limited, especially if you don't really understand your partner's or spouse's pain and the best ways to manage it. Nevertheless, there may be more options available to improve matters than you realise. A good place to start would be to read this book and to discuss it with your spouse or partner.

Spouses and partners of our patients have told us of the ways in which they have tried to deal with these types of issues. You may find some applicable to you or they may give you some ideas about the sorts of things you could try.

1 **Encourage your spouse or partner.** Allow your partner to try doing things he or she hasn't been doing because of pain—it may be quicker and easier for you to do it but he or she needs to start doing these things again. Encourage your partner in this. Try to find opportunities to allow your partner to take the initiative in doing things for him- or herself, for the family and socially. Encourage your partner to practise the methods described in this book to manage the pain more effectively. Remember, a good way to encourage someone to do something is to praise them for their achievements (or their progress towards the agreed goals).

2 **Get involved with his or her program.** The exercises he or she will be doing are suitable for all people regardless of whether or not they have pain. Exercise together—exercising can be fun. Learn to use the relaxation technique as well—we all get stressed at times so it is a very useful tool for everyone. Have a look at the way you think—unhelpful thinking affects all of us at different times, The skills taught in this book for managing pain are life skills that apply to all people with or without pain.

3 **Deal with any issues of dependency**—in you or your spouse or partner. As your partner tries to practise the approach outlined in this book you may find him or her becoming less dependent on you. You may experience a loss of role to start with but it is important that you both talk about your feelings as this occurs. Take the opportunity to develop your own interests and increase independence yourself. Set goals as a couple or a family to increase socialising, family activities and holidays.

4 **Try to make time to talk together** about your partner or spouse's pain and how it has affected both of you and your relationship. You may have had to endure a lot to support your

partner or spouse through some quite difficult times. It would be surprising if it hadn't affected you or your relationship. When you feel the time is right it can help to talk with your spouse or partner about how you have felt and your impressions of the changes in your relationship through the period of his or her pain problem. Do it in a way that is not blaming or accusing but learn to express your feelings again (rather than feeling as if you have to bite your tongue all the time). You may even have felt guilty that because you weren't the one with the problem, you really shouldn't be complaining. On the other hand, you may have grown increasingly resentful of the amount of time and effort you have had to put into helping your spouse. You don't have to be a martyr, and it may not be good for your relationship for you to feel that you have to be a martyr. At some point it will be helpful to discuss how it has been for you.

5 **Try to deal with any issues that concern you over your sexual relationship.** Talk about sexual difficulties. Encourage each other to try different techniques and positions. Say what you do and don't find enjoyable and express your needs also. You are working on this as a couple. Be prepared to make mistakes but also be prepared to have fun and laugh together as you work things out. Be adventurous. Address issues as they arise—don't wait for resentment to build up to an argument. Investigate the many resources available in bookshops on relationship and sexual communication issues. Some of these texts are recommended at the end of this book.

6 **Work on re-establishing good communication skills** if there are long-standing difficulties in your relationship. This is an issue often raised by our patients when talking about such matters. If needing help, either attend some classes in the community or seek some professional assistance. You can do a lot by just starting to talk about things again. Try working it out together first but if necessary, your GP may advise you on professional assistance available.

For the children of people in chronic pain

For older children

By reading this book we hope you will have a better understanding of your parent's pain and the options for managing it. Equally, you may have seen how you and your parent can work together to minimise the impact their pain has on you and your relationship.

There are some general points that can be made:

1 **Try not to worry about your parent** or feel that you need to protect him or her. Remember, in most cases they will still be quite well.

2 **Try to recognise patterns of unpredictable behaviour**, which may have made you avoid your parent. Discuss the problem of pain and mood swings, and discuss possible ways of dealing with these times.

3 **Encourage your parent** to keep using the strategies learnt from this book. Most people in persisting pain find it hard to keep practising these strategies. Support and encouragement from their family can be very helpful in this aspect. You might even find it fun (and good for your health) to join in with their exercise program.

4 **Do things together, especially things you both enjoy.** This can also help them to feel normal and accepted. Naturally, the activities chosen should be achievable for them. This should be negotiated, but try to start well-within their capacity rather than going for the maximum. Success with a small goal is usually better than another failure at something too ambitious.

5 **Try to pay more attention to their successes,** as these will have been achieved despite pain. Try to play down attention to failures, other than to see what both of you can learn from these.

6 **Look for ways that you can be helpful around the home.** To avoid doing too much for him or her (which they can find demeaning), try to negotiate which tasks you could do and which tasks they could manage.

For younger children

Younger children should be repeatedly reminded that their mother/father is well. They should be helped to understand that their parent is not dying and can still do most things around the home. It should be emphasised that many adults have these sorts of problems. However, they should be told that it is very unlikely that they will get the same problem when they are older. They can also be told that the problem can go away at times. In some cases it may be necessary to reassure the children that their parent's pain is not their fault—even when they aggravate their pain after a session of play or an argument with the children.

It should also be mentioned (as calmly and reassuringly as possible) that their parent does have some limits, and these should be pointed out only when necessary rather than drawing too much attention to them. Keep more emphasis on the things that are possible. As much as possible you should try to do as many normal things with your child as you can manage, even if you have to modify how you do it. For example, you could try playing board games sitting at a table instead of on the floor.

To help to normalise these situations it can also help if the children are encouraged to join in with the exercises and relaxation sessions with their parent. This should be done as something that might be fun rather than as a type of treatment. Try to show affection with physical play, but work out how you can do that without getting too rough. Cuddles don't have to end up as a wrestle. In some activities you may need to warn them that at times you may have to stop earlier than they might want, but at least you will have had some fun together.

For parents of children with pain

Whether your child is eight or fifteen, there are things you can do to be supportive.

One thing that most of us seem to agree on with this group (as with all age groups) is to avoid the quick remedies—that latest idea in a recently published magazine or the newest 'cure' on television may sound good to you but your child needs encouragement to follow the strategies in this book. You can play a major role here.

Perhaps a natural response for most parents will be to take over your child's responsibilities around the home. However, this requires careful handling as it is important that they retain a sense of achievement and independence despite their pain. They may not be able to do all the things you would like to see them doing, but it is often helpful to at least allow them a chance to try tasks and to learn to manage them, even if they don't do them perfectly. You have probably employed this strategy already in relation to many activities when they were younger.

Talk about the pain problem and explore with them possible ways of managing it—as outlined in the book, but try to avoid simply telling them what to do as that can often rile them, and undermine their own sense of competence. Be prepared to move on to other topics of conversation. Find shared interests and grow closer without focusing on pain.

If your child is younger you may have felt helpless and frustrated by the problem. You may have felt shut out because your partner has been more involved in treatment seeking for your child. Again, get involved with your child in normal activities.

> Take the example we mentioned earlier of Robyn. Robyn was 15 years old, and confined to a wheel chair due to a back injury caused by playing sport. She was taking excessive amounts of morphine. Her mother, a nurse, was very involved in seeking treatment for her daughter. Her father worked long hours. With Robyn's pain problem, he felt shut out and helpless to do anything. Tension escalated between father and daughter.
>
> When Robyn attended a pain management program her father was involved in driving her, a half-hour journey or more each way for three weeks. She was able to tell her father about the program as they travelled. Their relationship improved as he learnt more and she was able to show she was managing the problem independently. Their relationship is now much closer.

The teenage years are typically a difficult time, for both the teenagers and their parents, even without chronic pain. Having chronic pain can certainly add to the many stressors faced by children in this period.

Take the case of Jenny. Jenny had taken regular school holidays in an area of Australia where the mosquito borne Ross River Fever was prevalent. Over a period of time when she was about 15 years old she developed generalised aching in her muscles and stiff, sore joints. Of course, this coincided with a time when she was working and studying hard at school, and had episodes when she became quite tense and suffered headaches.

Nevertheless, she was able to continue playing netball and attending school. She just had pain in her arms when writing for long periods. Blood tests revealed that she had been exposed to the Ross River Fever. Knowing that this could be the cause of her symptoms was helpful, but there was no treatment to stop the symptoms. To some extent Jenny still felt that her condition had not been taken seriously, and that the doctor was uncaring and had virtually told her to go away and live with the symptoms.

In reality, the advice that Jenny received was similar to the advice you have read about in this book on accepting that despite all the advances in medical science many illnesses are still not curable. In these cases, how much the patient succeeds in accomplishing their goals in life will depend largely on how well they put the types of strategies described in this book into practice.

Fortunately, Jenny's mother encouraged her to follow this advice and did not keep pursuing more medical advice, even though there were some difficult times when Jenny felt she was not being taken seriously. Eventually Jenny's symptoms settled, although she did describe increases in her pain when she had additional demands on her time. Jenny is now 27 years old, she has successfully completed a university degree, in the midst of which she married and had two children. She now runs her own business as well as sharing the care of her home and children with her husband. Jenny still

has periods when she has muscle and joint pains, but she is confident that she is able to cope with them.

Interacting with others when you are in pain is often an added
stress. That is especially true when your pain is there most or all of
the time. Still, it is an issue which can't be avoided. If you can interact with those around you effectively, they can provide an
extremely valuable source of support. This can really help to lift
some of the load off your shoulders and improve your quality of
life—as well as their's. On the other hand, if your interactions with
others are often a problem then it is likely to make your pain that
much harder to manage. While no two people in pain will have
identical problems in their relationships with others, you can still
learn from the experiences of others. The material presented in this
chapter could help to give you some fresh ideas about your own
relationships. Of course, ideas may not be enough to help you deal
with these issues, but they might get you started. For many people,
it would also be worthwhile to seek the help of a trained counsellor, psychologist, or social worker.

Dealing With Flare-Ups and Set-Backs

Most people with chronic pain report their pain varies in intensity through the day, often depending on what they've been doing. If you have been using the ADAPT approach regularly you should have fewer flare-ups than previously, but they will still happen.

At times, your pain may get quite intense and difficult to bear, but it will often settle within a few hours. However, from time to time your pain may flare-up for a few days or even longer. No matter how long the increased pain lasts, you may have trouble keeping up your activities and exercises.

How long such flare-ups or set-backs last and how much trouble they cause will strongly influenced by the ways in which you deal with them.

You could simply wait till it happens, then stop everything, start taking pain killers or tranquillisers again, tell yourself the ADAPT approach hasn't worked, call the doctor out, and retire to bed for as long as it lasts. But what would be the likely result of that approach?

You probably don't need to think about it very long at this stage, but it is hard to see how that approach would really help, especially if it keeps being repeated.

On the other hand, if you accept that such temporary set-backs or flare-ups are bound to happen sooner or later, **you could work out a plan well in advance** and then put it into practice as soon as you become concerned about it.

There probably isn't a "best way" of dealing with set-backs or flare-ups that will work for everyone. But, by trying out different ways of dealing with set-backs you will eventually work out a plan that works best for you. Some basic strategies could help you to get started.

We have found it helpful to take this in stages. When your pain flares-up initially you won't really know how long the flare-up will last (even though you may start to think it could last forever). In most cases the flare-up will not last more than a day or so. In these cases that is all you need to get through. So, your initial strategies should be based on dealing with that period.

In other cases, the flare-up may go on for several days. That will mean you have to plan to deal with it over that time.

On the next page is an outline of a basic plan for dealing with the initial flare-up stage.

When your pain flares-up – a brief checklist

1) **STOP AND THINK** – What's happening? (clarify the problem)
   - Have I been overdoing something?
   - What can I do now – what are my options?
   - Work out a plan.

2) **IF POSSIBLE, TAKE YOUR TIME BEFORE REACTING**
   - Reacting without thinking (panic) could make things worse.
   - Identify any negative, unhelpful thoughts and instead think of other, more helpful ways of looking at the situation

3) **THINGS YOU COULD TRY**
   - Stop what you have been doing – **have a short break**. Look for something else to do for a while (eg: lie down briefly, go for a walk, do some stretch exercises).
   - **Relaxation – calm yourself** – spend a couple of minutes (or more) practising your relaxation technique.
   - **Use your desensitising technique – calmly focus your**

mind on the pain. Let it be there, don't try to push it away or block it. Remember, it's just activity in your nerves, and you are OK – it's not harming you.

- **Identify any negative thoughts – be realistic**. Thinking the worst never helps, instead you can remind yourself of more realistic and helpful thoughts."I know I can't make my pain go away completely, but I can cope with it". "I've coped with this pain before, I can do it again". "Even when it gets really bad I know it won't stay like that".
- **You might have to change some of your plans for the day**. You may have to pace things more for the rest of the day. What are your priorities – what can be left?

4) **THINGS TO AVOID**
   - **Carrying on without thinking** ("I'll just get this finished, then I'll stop").
   - **Over-reacting (catastrophising)** – you'll only get more upset.
   - **Stopping everything** and retiring to bed for the day – this might seem a good idea at the time, but is a long rest the answer?
   - **Taking pain killers** – an occasional one is OK, but they usually don't work as well as you'd like. There are drawbacks too – side effects and the risk of getting into a habit of using them to enable you to overdo things – not a sustainable option.
   - **Calling the doctor out** – you know by now that unless you have a new problem, there's not much he/she can do at these times (except give you more medication).

5) **WHEN THE PAIN STARTS TO EASE** review how you coped this time.
   - What can you learn from this episode?
   - What do you like about what you did?

- Recognise your achievements – praise yourself for coping as well as you did
- What could you do better next time?
- Check how well you have been pacing activities – could you do better?

If your pain flare-up continues for more than a day or so, then in addition to following the checklist on the last page you may need to take more comprehensive action. The points mentioned here could also be helpful if you have simply stopped doing the program due to something else, like an illness.

When things start going wrong for more than a day or so we call that a set-back because your daily activities may be significantly disrupted.

1) GET IN EARLY

The earlier you identify a set-back, the easier it will be for you to deal with it. Keeping some sort of record of your exercise practise or weekly activity goals could help you to pick up early signs of a set-back (such as starting to miss sessions or avoiding certain activities). On the other hand, you or those around you may start to notice you are wanting to rest more or to avoid going out. Use signs like these to put your set-back plan into operation (don't wait till you are having real trouble before acting).

You may also notice that set-backs tend to happen at certain times or in certain (high risk) situations, such as shopping in the week before Christmas or when the family visit you for the weekend. If you can see one of these times coming up, it could help to work out a plan to deal with it (e.g. spread out your tasks, get others to help, leave out unimportant tasks for the time being, explain to those around you that from time to time you will need to take short rest breaks to help you get through the day, etc.).

2) REASSURE YOURSELF

Periods of increased pain happen to most people with chronic

pain every now and then. Sometimes they last only a few hours, but at other times it may be a matter of days or even weeks. They may happen for no clear reason or they may be due to something you have overdone. One reason you could overlook may be after you have stopped your activity and exercise programme for a while (like during a holiday or while you have been in bed with the flu'). One thing you can be pretty sure of, though, is that depending on your condition, unless you've done something fairly dramatic (like fall down the stairs) the increased pain will not be due to some extra damage you've done to yourself.

3)   IF POSSIBLE, WORK OUT WHY

Review what may have led up to the set-back (or flare-up of pain). This could give you a guide to the best way to deal with the situation.

If you have been overdoing something and you are still doing it, you have a choice to make. Either carry on (and just accept that you will have to try to cope with the consequences later) or cut-back (stop what you're doing – try something else in a different position, do some relaxing, do some stretch exercises, etc. – then go back to what you were doing, but at a slower pace or with more breaks, if possible).

If you think the set-back (or flare-up) is due to what you have been doing over the last week, you could try to learn from it (and next time pace yourself more or do it differently). At the same time, you should pace your activities more today as well or do fewer things – and if you find some exercise is making things worse, do less of them for a day or two – then gradually pace them up again. **But don't stop everything!**

If you can't identify the cause of your flare-up, you will still face a choice – either carry on as if nothing has happened (but be ready to change if things continue getting worse) or cut back on your exercises and other activities for two or three days till the flare-up eases, then gradually pace them up again [this may take more than a week or two in some cases]. We recommend that you cut back your exercises by a reasonable amount – say, 50% on all exercises.

If the flare-up continues for more than a week or so, you may need to have a close look at how you've been doing things (overdoing repeatedly? not watching your posture?) or what you've been doing (too much of one activity, such as sitting?). You may also need to cut back on most of your exercises and activities (re-set your baselines for them) – then gradually pace them up again over a few weeks. This will take time and patience, but remember you did it just like this when you started the ADAPT programme. Remind yourself you are not back at square one, because now you know how to get out of it.

4) REMEMBER YOUR COPING STRATEGIES
Check if you are catastrophising about the set-back. **Are you thinking or reacting in a positive, realistic, helpful way?** It is alright to be concerned and careful, but worry and desperation don't help. Consider what you can do, what you did the last time you felt like this or were in this position. What seemed to help? What didn't help? What options are there? **It might help to re-read some sections of this handbook** to refresh your memory on ways of coping.

Are you getting tense or wound up? **Remember your relaxation and desensitisation techniques.**

5) BE FLEXIBLE BUT REALISTIC
Depending on how things are going, **you may need to change your plans** as the set-back persists, such as stop one exercise completely for a few days or put off a planned outing. But remember, most of the things you try to deal with the set-back will not work 100% (very few things are 100% successful). But that doesn't mean you should stop doing them completely. At these difficult times it is especially important to try to **keep a balanced view on things**. So, if the relaxation technique doesn't seem to help as much, don't stop doing it – at least by doing it you are doing what you can and it will be a lot better than getting into a panic over the set-back. You may need to remind

yourself that you've survived difficult times before and, if you can hang on now, you will get through the present trouble.

6) HELP FROM OTHERS

Normally, you will want the people around you (at home, work, etc.) to stand back and let you get on with things, unless you specifically ask for their help. However, when you're having a set-back, it can help to explain to your family or friends (or co-workers, etc.) what is happening (trying not to sound alarmist) – what you will be trying to do to deal with the problem – and, most importantly, what you would like them to do (or not to do). By making these points as clearly as possible (but not in a demanding way), you will help the people around you to help you rather than hinder you. At the same time they will be reassured and will find it easier to understand what you're going through (remember no one can read minds, no matter how well they know you).

If you're finding it hard to cope by yourself, even with helpful friends or family, you could always try going to see your doctor to discuss the situation with him or her. Sometimes, they might think of something you've overlooked. Maybe it is time that you were referred to a multidisciplinary pain clinic for assessment and help with your pain?

7) WHEN IT'S OVER

It's natural that you would just want to forget about it, but **we recommend that you spend a bit of time reviewing how you dealt with each set-back or flare-up**. This can help you to learn ways of coping better next time and, perhaps, ways of preventing some future set-backs.

Reinforce your achievements – what did you like about the way you coped? Did you deal with the set-back better than last time? What could you do better next time?

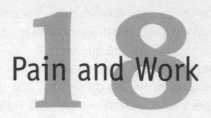

Pain and Work

Summary:

Staying at work despite chronic pain is generally a good idea. There are many positives for us in working. Usually, working despite chronic pain requires some flexibility from both the worker and the workplace as some adjustments will be needed. But with goodwill on both sides, and good problem-solving strategies, most people with chronic pain can find useful employment. This chapter outlines some of the strategies that can be used to make work possible when you have chronic pain.

Pain doesn't have to stop you working. In fact, many people with chronic pain continue to work and to find satisfaction in their work, even if they have to modify the ways in which they work. Understandably, however, many of the people who develop chronic pain do find it difficult to maintain their jobs as before. They may find aspects, such as the amount of sitting, standing or lifting, too difficult to keep up all day, even if they can do it for short periods. Some find that their employer is unwilling or unable to assist by agreeing to modify the demands of the job or to allow some flexibility. In these cases, the person with chronic pain may have to consider seeking more suitable employment. Some people with chronic pain appear to struggle on as they don't want to lose their job or they fear they will be unable to find anything better elsewhere and they need the money. In these cases, we often find that people in this position do little else than work then "crash" when they get home at the end of the day. Their home and social lives may bear the brunt of the drive to stay at work.

It is also true that many people with chronic pain find they cannot continue to work and give up hope of ever getting back to work. Finding a job that you can do without aggravating your pain so much that you can't do anything when you get home is often difficult. In general, the type of work (especially how physically-demanding it is) can influence your chances of returning to work or keeping your existing job. Interestingly, however, evidence from the New South Wales WorkCover Authority suggests that it is not just the nature of the job that is important. For example, the proportion of injured workers who haven't returned to work within 6-months of injury is very similar for manual and office workers (17% versus 16%).

Whether or not someone returns to work after an injury depends on many issues apart from the nature of the job. For example, the availability of a suitable job, the skills of the worker (clearly, the more skills you have the better your chances will be), and the willingness of an employer to take on someone with a history of injury (especially if they have had a workers compensation claim in the past). Some, of course, do not want to return to work and may settle for improving their quality of life at home.

Despite the obstacles, many people with chronic pain do return to work. We have tried to learn from their experiences.

Peter was a classic example. Peter's job was at risk. Attending our program and showing that he could be reliable at work was Peter's last chance, and Peter was very keen to keep his job. Therefore he was committed to attending for our 3 week program. However, his attitude and behaviour in the first week made it clearly evident that he didn't really believe any of this could make any difference.

However, to his credit, he persevered and attempted to at least trial the strategies. Early in the 3rd week, when Peter was making significant gains in coping with his pain, and was seeing improvements in his personal life at home, Peter said to us. "You know, I really didn't believe any of this could help in the first week". We looked in mock surprise and said, "Oh, is that so, Peter?" "Was it that obvious?" he asked.

But Peter did apply the strategies, and was extremely proud of himself, and pleased with the significant progress he had made. A meeting was arranged with the relevant people from Peter's workplace and he returned to work confidently following the program, believing that he had the skills required to satisfy the demands of the workplace, as well as his personal life.

This chapter outlines some of things we have learned from experiences like Peter's. As with the other complex issues covered in this book we would recommend that you seek out professional assistance if you are not confident about dealing with this area on your own. In every country there are public and/or private agencies that can help people return to work after injury. Initially, most injured workers will be effectively guided by their doctor. But other health professionals, as well as employers, can also help. Access to different services varies between countries and you may need to get information on what help is available in your country. Usually, this information can be obtained from your doctor, employer, union or Government agencies. In the UK, for example, the offices of the Department of Work and Pensions (DWP) should be able to give you advice on available rehabilitation services. A recent innovation in the UK has been the creation of the position of Personal Adviser in the DWP as a means of providing disabled people with advice and help in finding suitable assistance for overcoming the many obstacles faced when attempting to remain at work or to find new jobs.

It is important to realise that while your doctor is able to advise you on the best treatments for your injuries and pain, he/she may have limited knowledge and expertise when it comes to return to work issues. You are likely to need additional help, especially if you are having (or have had) trouble returning to work. This is especially true if you have been out of work for many weeks or months.

We recommend that you discuss with your doctor the sorts of difficulties or obstacles you are facing in returning to work, but also say that you didn't expect him/her to solve these problems for you. Instead, you could ask his/her help in finding out who could provide assistance in this area. It would be ideal if you and your doctor could work in a cooperative way with whoever is able to help you in your efforts to return to work.

In many cases, returning to one's previous type of work may not be realistic. You may need to consider looking for ways of retraining or learning new skills to help you become employable again. Most countries offer training in practical work skills through technical colleges, but available courses are likely to differ from place to place. You will need to do some asking around to find out what is available near you.

Things to consider about work and pain

(1) Do you want to work? This may seem an odd question, but there is little point in going through the motions of trying to work if you really don't want to. How could you know? At present you may not feel like working, but who knows, this feeling may change as you apply this programme and get more confident about what you can do. Re-examining the chapter on setting goals could help you to work out your priorities here.

(2) Is it realistic for anyone in pain to work? In general, the answer is yes. As mentioned earlier many people work despite pain. Providing they can make the necessary adjustments (such as pacing activities, modifying postures and minimising difficult tasks), many people have returned to work after injury despite persisting pain. Naturally, this is usually best done by negotiating with your employer about what you can manage and what assistance or accommodations you require, at least to begin with. Over time, as you build up your tolerances these arrangements can change.

One patient who attended our programme at the hospital, for example, was taking over 400mg of morphine a day and was unable to perform her clerical job. Nevertheless, her employer said he was willing to take her back if she could attend reliably and build up her hours over time. After attending the programme with us she was able to cease her use of morphine and had paced up her exercises to the point where she felt ready to return to work for a couple of hours a day. The employer agreed and a return to work plan was arranged. The plan involved her gradually pacing up her time at work, starting with two 2-hour blocks a day for three days a week (working every second day). Her 2-hour work blocks were separated by an hour or so when she would do her exercises at a nearby gym. At the time of writing (about 16 months since she completed the programme), this patient is still working (now 5 hours a day, 5 days a week), and she has not taken anything for her pain for over a year. She is happy with this work level as it still leaves time for other things she likes to do and she doesn't burn herself out at work. We believe that one of the key reasons for this lady's success was the willingness of her employer to compromise and find ways of helping (as opposed to blocking).

A large study in the state of Michigan in the United States of America also found that those employers who found ways to help their injured workers return to work tended to have better success in return to work rates than those who did not. So, when an employer says they have "no light duties" or "you have to be 100% fit before you can come back to work", it seems to us that such employers are not really trying to help someone return to work. Remember, most people who work are not that fit.

(3) Using problem-solving. Working despite pain is clearly an area which requires good problem-solving skills. Often the best solutions will not be ideal, but they may be better than not working at all. Re-read the chapter on problem solving (Chapter 15). One good example of this was a man who had been a truck driver when he was injured. A year or two later when his pain had not improved he attended our programme and, despite being quite despondent before it, he did pick himself up and when he returned home he managed to get a new job as a tour bus driver. He has kept this job for a couple of years now and he looks a different person to the one who attended our programme. When we asked him how he managed to keep driving with his painful back, he said he had worked out that if he stopped the bus every hour or so (to give the tourists an opportunity to get off the bus and take a look about) he could keep his pain under control. So he had found a job that he had the skills to do (as a former truck driver) and he could still pace his sitting so that he didn't overdo it and stir up his pain.

(4) Dealing with stress. A number of studies have shown that workers who are dissatisfied with their jobs and feel stressed or unhappy at work, tend to have more trouble in returning to work after injury. On the other hand, some recent treatment studies in Scandinavia have shown that if injured workers with back problems learn effective ways of dealing with stress they have more success in staying at work. Have another look at the chapters on Challenging Ways of Thinking About Pain (Chapter 11), and Stress and Problem-Solving (Chapter 15). If you find your work is made harder by stress, then you may be able to improve how you are dealing with it. This may also help you stay at work.

However, it is also true that other people at work will often be part of the problem. It could be your boss or other workers or colleagues. Have another look at the chapter on Interacting With Those Around You (Chapter 16). This could help to prepare you to deal with others at work more effectively. This is also an area where a rehabilitation provider should be able to assist you and help you to negotiate a reasonable arrangement with your boss, as well as other colleagues. If these problems are related to your not being able to do as much as you used to do, due to your pain, it might help to show them this book.

Remember what you were like before your pain became chronic? How would you have looked at someone like you now? Maybe you could discuss this with your colleagues or workmates?

Some people with chronic pain have told us that they looked for ways of "trading" some of their duties with others, so that they did some of the tasks the others normally did, while the others picked up some of their more difficult tasks. Naturally, this can be awkward and this could be an area where the help of a trained rehabilitation provider could make a big difference.

(5) Alternatives to work. Whatever has caused your pain, it is helpful to return to your normal activities as soon as possible, to avoid becoming depressed and despondent, as well as disabled. This includes returning to some sport or fitness activity, even a simple walking program, preferably with some company. Your local community services, council or library can often be a good source of information on what is available in your district.

Another way of gradually resuming some fulfilling activities is to do some voluntary work. Most local councils will be able to give you information about what is available. If you are not ready (or don't wish) to return to paid work just yet, then doing some voluntary work can be a first step. This can not only help you to feel useful, but also it can give you some useful "on the job" training and help you to get up to "freeway speed" and ready to return to more demanding work.

Ergonomics

For a lot of people, a large part of their day is spent in one position. This may be at a desk in front of a computer or studying, driving long distances, standing at a work bench or any number of positions. Or maybe you are only doing activities for relatively short periods, such as ironing. Whatever you are doing, it is important that you look at your work environment and make sure that it is as comfortable as possible for you. If you would like more advice on the best layout for your office or work-space you could consider consulting an ergonomist. Ergonomists are people who have special training in this area and they can be a good source of ideas for what might help you.

An example of sitting at a computer is given here. Sometimes it

Sitting at a Computer

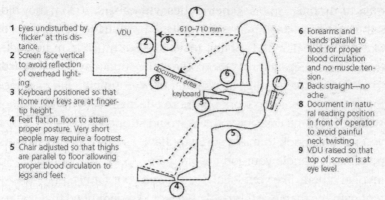

1 Eyes undisturbed by 'flicker' at this distance.
2 Screen face vertical to avoid reflection of overhead lighting.
3 Keyboard positioned so that home row keys are at fingertip height.
4 Feet flat on floor to attain proper posture. Very short people may require a footrest.
5 Chair adjusted so that thighs are parallel to floor allowing proper blood circulation to legs and feet.

6 Forearms and hands parallel to floor for proper blood circulation and no muscle tension.
7 Back straight—no ache.
8 Document in natural reading position in front of operator to avoid painful neck twisting.
9 VDU raised so that top of screen is at eye level.

Poor posture limits the circulation of the blood, puts pressure on the heart, and reduces the flow of nutrients to the muscles and the brain. Have you considered that even when you are at rest, your body is expending a great deal of energy just to stop you collapsing under the force of gravity?

means making some changes to the area in which you are going to work, but in the long run it is worth it.

However adjusting equipment alone will not be all that is required. It is important to assess your work flow and the activities you are performing and to plan them so that you can make regular changes in your position using pacing to gradually do more. An awareness of your posture and the ability to change your posture remains essential to optimise work safety.

Sofia was a good example of these principles.

Sofia was suffering neck pain following a motor vehicle accident. She was a school teacher and was keen to resume marking exam papers. However, the fixed posture involved with reading and writing was a problem. She was able to use a sloping desk board and had adjusted her sitting posture. She had also been working on building up her tolerance for using her arms in a fixed position. As a result, she had learnt that there was a time limit that she could sit and mark papers. Therefore she set her timer and took a short break and changed her position. Eventually she found that she could actually mark more papers, and not suffer so greatly at the end.

In conclusion

Clearly, there are many issues involved in returning to work while still in pain or staying at work despite pain. In some cases it is likely that the demands of the job will be too much to manage. In these cases, consideration about alternative options is clearly wise. In other cases, it may just be a matter of re-examining the nature of the work and trying to work out more effective ways of managing. Whichever is the case for you, we would strongly recommend that you use this book to make sure you have as many of the skills as possible to handle your job despite pain. It can also be helpful to involve others, like your local doctor, and your family. But, consistent with the theme of this book, we would recommend that you try not to let pain stop you achieving your return to work goals.

Pain Self-Management for Seniors

O ver the last 5 years we have been testing the methods outlined in this book with people aged over 65 years (and up to 90) who were seeking help for their chronic pain. We have found that these methods can help older people, but as with younger people, you have to do them regularly for several weeks before you will see benefits. But there are some differences between younger and older people with pain that are worth knowing about.

On the positive side, our research (and research by others) has found that older people with chronic pain are generally less distressed about it than younger people. The older people seemed to be more accepting of their chronic pain and realize they do have to learn to live with it.

On the negative side, older people with chronic pain are more likely to have other conditions as well (like osteoarthritis, blood pressure problems, heart disease, respiratory illnesses, and so on). These other conditions do need to be considered when planning your pain management program, so we suggest you discuss your plans with your doctor. This applies especially to your exercises and medications. A few key points should help older people make best use of the book.

Medications

Many people over 65 years of age will be taking medications for medical conditions other than pain, and they often want to avoid taking pain medication if possible. One of the important points here is the risk of adverse interactions between your pain medications and other medications (like drowsiness, stomach and bowel problems). But it is important not to add or change medications without discussing it with your doctor first. If you do want to minimise your pain medications, the methods described in the book can help.

Remember, for many older people staying active and independent are more important goals than waiting for pain relief. So, exercises can help here.

Exercises

The chapters on **setting goals** (Chapter 7) and **pacing** (Chapter 8) were found to be very helpful. So, developing a brief activity upgrading and exercise plan is a good place to start.

As we mentioned in the exercise chapter, the exercises are to help you get moving (and to keep moving), rather than to relieve pain. The basic message is: *if you are active but in pain you will have a better quality of life than someone who is inactive and in pain.*

Several of the exercises described in the book will be too demanding for many older people and you should start by selecting the ones you think you can manage. If you can discuss it with a physiotherapist that is better still.

Many older people are not comfortable with gyms, so doing these exercises in a room with enough space at home is fine. Doing the exercises with another family member or a group of friends can help to make them more fun.

Doing exercises with a group in a heated pool is also popular with older people and worth trying. But as we don't live in the water it is important to exercise on land too.

For resistance work you can use either the commercially available rubber stretch-bands (sometimes called *Thera-bands*) or light weights (like barbells) that can be bought at sports stores. Alternatively, put small tins of food in a light bag and use them.

Do try to use your exercise chart from the book and to pre-set the exercise quotas at least a day (or week) before you do them. Check them off on your exercise chart as you achieve your quotas. Gradually, you should try to pace up your quotas as we discussed in Chapter 8 (on pacing). Show your exercise chart to your doctor (and physiotherapist, nurse, or family members) every few weeks so they can see what you're able to do.

Goal setting

Try to start with small, achievable goals, like walking to a neighbour's place or sitting through a meal. Then gradually aim higher, for more ambitious goals that you'd like to achieve. As always, pacing is essential for sustained improvement in functioning.

Keep a chart for recording your goals and tick them off as you achieve them – that is usually quite rewarding. Remember, it is you who has done it and you've done it now despite your pain.

Thought management and relaxation

Unhelpful thoughts about pain and other problems do make managing pain harder. Thoughts like "I can't go on" or "I can't cope with this" will make anyone feel hopeless, even if they seem realistic. These sorts of 'catastrophic' thoughts are still just thoughts. We don't have to go along with them, but it helps to recognise you're having them in order to manage them.

To manage unhelpful thoughts we suggest you try to put them to one side (without fighting them or trying to stop them – that can even encourage them). Instead, try to focus on what you want to do – your immediate goal, like getting out of bed or have a short walk. Then work out how you'll do it, accepting the pain will be there but it doesn't have to stop you. Plan your activity and remember to pace yourself, a bit at a time.

If you are feeling stressed or worried you might also like to try the relaxation technique as well (see Chapter 12). This means using your breathing to let go a bit of tension each time you breathe out. The aim of this is to help you manage, not to take the pain away.

We recommend you use the relaxation technique while you are doing other things, including exercising. This means just letting go as you breathe out while you exercise or walk or whatever. You may not become as relaxed as you might in a quiet place but it will help you to stay as calm as possible in a stressful place.

The attentional technique of desensitizing we describe (Chapter 13) is also worth trying along with the relaxation technique. It's a bit like confronting your fears. Just calmly go into your pain sensations with your mind with as little reaction as possible, observe the sensations without trying to change them or even think about them. See what happens instead of thinking about it. It is intended to help you lessen the impact of pain rather than lessen the pain. Treat it as an experiment, but you will need to practice it several times a day (and at night in bed) to get the most out of it.

Communicating with others

As we discussed in Chapter 16, it is helpful to tell people you're close to about your pain management plan, so they will understand when you are pacing your activities and can encourage you to keep working on it. Explaining your program to them (even get them to read parts of the book) can also help to reduce their worries about you and concerns they may have about your pain not going away.

Maintenance

A key finding in our research was that other events in your life will often get in the way of keeping to your pain management program. Events like getting a cold or another illness, as well as extra demands from family or friends (who might also get sick or have some infirmity). These disruptions are to be expected and you can only try to work around them as best you can. If you can't do your exercises for a week or so, that is OK. Just try to get back to them as soon as possible, but remember to start with a little less than you were doing before the stoppage, then pace yourself back up.

Of course, even if you can't manage your exercises you can

often still work on your pacing and thought management, as well as the relaxation technique.

Finally, try to give yourself regular pats on the back for your efforts. You're still trying even if you can't be perfect. No one else can either.

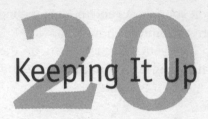

Keeping It Up

Long-term success with this programme will depend on your ability to continue using the skills and techniques you have learnt.

Follow-up interviews with ex-ADAPT patients have clearly shown that those who have done best in the long-term are the ones who have kept up their pacing, relaxation and fitness exercises, as well as the various coping strategies they learnt at ADAPT. That is not to say it is always easy (of course, it isn't), but it does show the benefit of continuing to use the skills and approaches learnt on the programme.

Once you've succeeded in making changes, and you're achieving many of your goals, the next question will be how to keep up your progress. When you first started this programme, you will probably have found that family, friends or your doctor provided plenty of support and encouragement. But once you're on your way, they may not have as much time to help. Alternatively, they may feel you don't really need that much support any longer. However, you may find it quite hard to keep things going – things like staying off the pain killers, keeping up your exercises and working towards your long-term goals. This is especially true if you have any setbacks or stop your programme for a while due to something like the flu'. Once again, it would seem a good idea to think about these issues and ways of dealing with it before you have to face them.

What problems do you think you might have in maintaining the changes you have made and how could you deal with them?

1) No support or encouragement at home?

Naturally, it can help a great deal if your family or friends are able to reinforce your efforts with support and encouragement. However, this doesn't always happen. Your family or friends may not help because either they don't understand your pain problem and don't know what they can do to help or, for some reason, they are unwilling or unable to help. How could you deal with this?

Discuss it with them. If it seems they don't understand or don't know how to help, perhaps you could discuss the programme with them, get them to read this book (or bits of it), or ask them to discuss the programme with you and your doctor.

You will probably need to explain to your friends or family what you are trying to do and tell them **exactly** how they can help. For example, perhaps they could join in your exercise sessions or you might like them to take over one of your responsibilities while you do your exercises. Sometimes they might help you most by leaving you alone at the times you specify so you can get on with your own activities or exercises. Whatever the case, discussing your plans with them and making it clear what you would like from them will often help to avoid misunderstandings and possible conflict.

Deal with expectations. It is quite likely that your friends or family will have become used to the way you were before you started the programme. As a result they may need time to adjust to the ways in which you have changed. They may just expect you to go back to the way you were before the programme and so act as if nothing has changed – something you might find upsetting after all your efforts. Or they may expect too much of you too soon and not understand that it may still take some time before you are as active as you (and they) would like you to be.

If it seems your family or friends are unwilling or unable to help, it may still help to clarify this with them so that you know where you stand and what to expect from them.

Reinforce yourself. If, for whatever reason, you don't have anyone to encourage you it is important to do it yourself – as was discussed in the section on making changes. In other words, reinforce yourself for your gains. But, remember not to rely on the same one or two reinforcers all the time – try to add to your list of reinforcers, and use them all. Occasionally, you could even give yourself a really big reinforcer, such as a holiday, a meal in a restaurant or some new clothes – providing, of course, that you achieved your goals first.

2) A tendency to put off doing things or forget?

No doubt you will agree that if you make only vague plans to carry on with the programme (or "just wait and see how it goes") you probably won't carry them out. For example, if you say you will try to keep up your exercises every day but don't work out how, you will probably find yourself putting off doing them.

Make specific plans. You will be much more successful if you can make some specific plans about how and when you are going to do your activities and exercises. For example, you could decide to do your exercises at a set time each day. By doing your exercises at a specific time and place, such as in front of the TV news at 6pm, you will find that after a week or two it has become as much a habit as cleaning your teeth before bed at night (or whenever you clean them). Similarly, if one of your goals is to attend something like an adult education class you could easily keep putting-off finding out when it started. Making a specific plan to do it on a set day (and even writing this down in your diary or on a kitchen notice board) will help you to make sure you do it.

Use reminders. It can often help to use specific reminders to help you remember what you have to do. For example, if you have trouble remembering to relax when you're sitting in your car, it could help to place a sticky label on the steering wheel where you'll catch sight of it. Similarly, if you have trouble remembering how to use the vacuum cleaner properly (with the best posture), placing a label on the vacuum cleaner could remind you each time you go to use it.

On the other hand, you can simply try to get into the habit of associating a particular activity with a certain time or place. You can do this by performing the activity as often as possible at that time or place. For example, doing your exercises at the same time or place each day, or checking your posture each time you sit down (before doing anything else).

It can also help to reinforce yourself each time you remember to carry out your plans – it will make it easier to remember next time.

3) Other demands on your time?

It is quite likely that from time to time you will find you have to put your plans aside in order to deal with other demands on your time – things like requests from friends or family members to help them with something, or perhaps you may take a holiday or even get the flu'. At these times it may be quite impossible to keep up your exercises or working on some planned activity. This sort of temporary interruption shouldn't be a problem – when the interruption is over you should be able to get back to your own plans (though you may have to restart your exercises and some other activities at levels below what they were when you stopped).

However, if you find the other demands on your time seem to be going on too long you may need to re-think things. For example, you may need to sort out your priorities – what is more important to you: to leave things the way they are and to forget your exercises and goals, or to stop what you're doing and get back to your exercises and working towards your goals? If you don't want to give up either, then you will have to make some sort of compromise and find a middle way which allows you to do some of both.

Sometimes the issue may involve your friends or family and you may find it difficult to discuss the matter with them. If so, it may be worth spending a little time thinking about a good way to go about it. Reading a book on communication skills could help here. Of course, you might also like to discuss this issue with your doctor or clinical psychologist, or other health care provider.

Whatever you decide it is most important that you don't let things drift too long – the longer you leave your exercises and goals the harder it will be to get back to them.

Some points about the programme to keep in mind

1) Keep active – in as many areas of your daily life as possible. Especially in household chores, leisure or hobbies, family/social activities, exercise, work (paid or unpaid).

Remember: – use pacing and plan your days as much as possible to get a good balance of activity through the day and the week (try to avoid loading all your activities onto one part of the day or one day in the week and try to vary your activities – not too much sitting or standing at once).

2) Things to Avoid
- Too much resting.
- Relying on drugs (including alcohol) to help you cope.
- Thinking in negative, unrealistic and unhelpful ways.
- Thinking in unrealistically positive ways.
- Focussing on how much the pain hurts.
- Talking about the pain.

3) Deal with set-backs or lapses – (and learn from them). These are bound to happen at times. Learn from the ways you dealt with the last one and work out what you can do better next time. Read Chapter 18 (on dealing with set-backs and increased pain). Most importantly, don't let things just drift – do something about it!

4) Take the credit for your achievements. Only you know how difficult it is to live with pain. Others can help a bit, but in the end it is up to you. By taking the credit for your achievements you will improve your confidence in yourself and in your ability to cope with pain.

5) Encouragement from others. Family and friends can help in many ways. In particular they should:

- Acknowledge and praise your efforts and achievements (even if you are not always successful – who is?);
- Avoid asking about the pain (you can tell them when necessary);
- Avoid urging you on or pushing you to do things (it's up to you to do decide what you are going to do);
- Avoid doing things for you because of your pain (unless you ask first).

6) Working with your doctor.
Have another look at Chapter 5 on Working With Your Doctor. You shouldn't need to see him/her very often about your pain, but every now and then it can be helpful to let him/her know how you are managing. We recommend that you stay with one doctor as long as possible, as that will help your doctor to keep a consistent approach to managing your pain. You can also seek advice from your doctor from time to time if you hear about a "new" treatment or "breakthrough" for pain.

Final Check

Go back to the Introduction and have another look at how you would score yourself now on the Pain Management Strategies Checklist.

On items 1 and 2 if you score 3 or more you are doing quite well – give yourself some reinforcement (if less than 3, you still have some work to do).

On items 3 to 17, if you don't score any 2's, 3's or 4's you probably don't need to read this book again – for the time being. Give yourself another reinforcer.

If you still score 2, 3 or 4 on any of these items you should discuss it with your doctor. It might also help if you discussed it with a clinical psychologist or a physiotherapist with experience and training in cognitive-behavioural treatments. You should also consider asking to be referred to a multidisciplinary pain clinic or pain centre.

Glossary

Analgesics Medicines that are used to reduce or relieve pain.

Anxiety Feeling very troubled by worries or fears. Often accompanied by physical symptoms like sweating, feelings of tension, heart racing, difficulty breathing and dry mouth.

Catastrophising A tendency to think the worst about situations. Such thoughts are usually extreme and negative (for example, 'I'll never be able to do this'). These thoughts are generally unhelpful.

Cognitions Thoughts; ways of thinking; perceptions.

Cognitive behavioural therapy A type of psychological treatment which helps you to examine the ways you think and respond to certain problem situations in your life. Then the treatment focuses on helping you to learn more helpful ways of thinking and responding to these situations and others that you might face.

Complex regional pain syndrome Also known as reflex sympathetic dystrophy. May occur after an injury, particularly if a nerve is damaged. In addition to continuing pain there is one or more of the following symptoms: swelling, sweating and colour change which are present after the normal period of healing.

Coping strategies Thoughts and behaviours that are used to manage or cope with stressful situations, such as pain or demands made by other people.

Cordotomy Surgical interruption of nerve pathways in the spinal cord.

Depression In general, depression refers to feeling sad or despondent. It can be short-lived or be a pervading feeling that can last for months. At its most severe depression can be considered an illness, especially if it becomes debilitating. When more severe it can be accompanied by feelings of hopelessness, worthlessness, as well as loss of appetite and weight, disturbed sleeping, irritability, lethargy, and loss of interest in previously enjoyable aspects of life, including sex. If someone becomes very depressed and experiences the sorts of symptoms described here they should see their doctor. Such depressions place them at risk of suicide. Depression is treatable with both medications and cognitive behavioural therapy.

Discectomy Surgical removal of all or part of the intervertebral disc.

Facet joint Paired joints in the back that support and allow movement of the spine.

Intrathecal space Fluid filled space around the spinal cord and brain.

Kyphosis Excessive forward angulation of the spine.

Myofascial pain syndrome (also called fibrositis and myalgia). Usually characterised by areas of tenderness (sometimes called 'trigger points') across widespread areas of the body. People thought to have this syndrome usually report that passive stretch or strong voluntary contraction of their muscles is painful.

Nerve A part of the body that transmits electrical messages through the body. All instructions from the brain to the rest of the body are transmitted along nerves. All input to the brain, from the rest of the body, is transmitted along the nerves to different parts of the brain.

Neuropathic pain Pain that is associated with injury or disease of a nerve, the spinal cord or the brain. The pain is often described as being burning, shooting, stabbing or squeezing. In fact, any painful sensation that a person can experience may be described.

Neurotomy A procedure involving the cutting of a nerve.

Nociceptive pain This type of pain may be experienced after an injury to any part of the body. It is usually dull and aching. The pain is usually well localised—that is, in a well-defined area.

Opiate/Opioid Drugs that have an action like morphine.

Pain behaviours The ways in which people may behave when they are in pain. Common examples are making complaints about pain, taking analgesics, lying down during the day, rubbing the affected area of the body, grimacing, groaning, guarding the painful site, limping, using an aid such as a stick or a collar. These behaviours can also indicate to other people that the person is in pain.

Prolapsed intervertebral disc (commonly called a 'slipped disc') The disc doesn't actually slip. Rather, a tear may develop in the disc and some of the material inside the disc may seep out and put pressure on a spinal nerve, leading to pain.

Reflex sympathetic dystrophy See **Complex regional pain syndrome**.

Reinforcer A reward or acknowledgment of an achievement following something you have done. It is usually seen as something desirable, but its effect is to encourage the person to repeat the behaviour or action that led to the reinforcer, in the expectation that the reinforcer will be obtained again. If the behaviour is not repeated, the reinforcer was not very effective. Almost anything can be a reinforcer. It can be something tangible— such as a cup of coffee or a night out—or less obvious— like giving credit for an achievement or recognising an achievement. Simply achieving a goal can also be a reinforcer and an encouragement to keep going. The withdrawal of something unpleasant can also act as a reinforcer. This is called 'negative reinforcement'. Thus, if something eases your pain you will probably use it again (because it worked before). The reduction in pain is the negative reinforcer.

Retrolisthesis A backward slip of one vertebrae on top of another.

Rhizotomy Basically, cutting a spinal nerve root which carries a sensation.

Scoliosis A curve to the side of the spine that can develop in both children and adults.

Sciatica Pain in the back of thigh, leg and foot associated with a prolapsed intervertebral disc.

Slipped disc See **Prolapsed Disc**.

Spinal cord Specialised tissue consisting of nerve cells lying within the spine.

Spondylosis Damage to the spine from wear and tear.

Spondylolisthesis A forward slip of one vertebrae on top of another.

Trigger points Localised areas of increased tenderness in muscle.

Vertebra One of the bones that makes up the back.

Vertebral slip As the vertebrae sit on top of each other, a forward or backward slip may occur because of wear and tear or a break in one the stabilising bony arches in the back.

Visceral pain Injury or disease affecting the organs of the chest or 'stomach'. The pain is usually deep and dull, and can be difficult to localise.

Zygapophyseal joint See **Facet Joint**.

Appendix 1

Evidence of Effectiveness of ADAPT-type treatments

It is now accepted practice in health care that all treatments being offered to patients should have a reasonable amount of evidence to support their effectiveness. No treatment works for everyone, but it is reasonable that anyone considering a new treatment should know that the treatment works better than chance, or better than no treatment, for their sort of problem. In the field of chronic pain there are currently no curative treatments. Some treatments have been shown to relieve pain, but to date these have been only temporary effects. The most treatments can offer is some improvement in symptoms (such as pain severity) or reduced impact of the pain on the person and their lifestyle.

The ADAPT program is known as a cognitive behavioural treatment. As mentioned in Chapter 6 'Treatments for Chronic Pain', cognitive behavioural treatments for chronic pain are not aimed at the underlying cause of pain, but rather at reducing the impact of pain on the person and their daily activities. In particular, they address the person's emotional state, their range of daily activities, their sleep, and often their use of unhelpful medication or other passive treatments that can limit a person's ability to rehabilitate themselves. To some extent these treatments also address pain. If a person in persisting pain can find ways to limit the impact of pain on how they feel and their daily activities they will often say that while their pain is still present it doesn't bother them as much as it did when it was disrupting most areas of their life.

There are now more than 30 studies of cognitive behavioural treatments for chronic pain. Most of these studies have compared the treatment against either a group receiving no treatment or some standard treatment. However, it should be realised that when someone in chronic pain participates in a study of this sort of treatment they have already undergone many other treatments to no avail. In general, studies of cognitive behavioural treatments with chronic pain problems only use people in whom standard medical (mainly drug) treatments or surgery have been tried and failed or ruled out as inappropriate. So the question arises for all those who suffer from chronic pain and their doctors plus other therapists, what can a person do when they reach that point? A choice has to be made between going on as before or seeking another way. The approach outlined in this book represents an alternative to ongoing trials of passive treatments in people for whom they have not worked.

If passive treatments, whether it is analgesic drugs, surgery, chiropractic or faith healing, have helped and the person in pain is quite happy with the results then that is wonderful. They may not need to explore the approach described in this book. On the other hand, if that is not the case, this book describes an approach which has been demonstrated to be effective in achieving targeted outcomes in a number of countries. By 'targeted outcomes' we mean outcomes which the treatments were aiming for, rather than ones which they weren't. That is, cognitive behavioural pain management can achieve improved mood, increased activity levels, reduced use of unhelpful medication and reduced pain levels. But this treatment does not cure the underlying cause of chronic pain.

Review studies
Three major reviews of outcome studies published during 1990s reported solid support for the effectiveness of these treatments as a group with a range of chronic pain conditions. The actual components of each cognitive behavioural treatment do vary from study to study, as do the types of patients and their problems. Thus there is often variation in degree of outcomes achieved. In some ways this is a bit like different doses of the same drug having different degrees of effect. If you take too small a dose, the effect may be minimal. Best results may only be achieved with a large dose of the drug. Nevertheless, when the better studies of cognitive behavioural treatments for chronic pain are lumped together and their effects are compared with common alternatives, the overall trend is clear. These treatments are effective. See:

Flor, H., Fydrich, T. and Turk, D.C. (1992) Efficacy of multidisciplinary pain treatment centres: a meta-analytic review *Pain* 49, 221–230.

McQuay, H., Moore, Eccleston, C., Morley, S. and Williams, A.C.deC. (1997) *Health Technology Assessment, 1997: Systematic Review of Outpatient Services for Chronic Pain Control*

Morley, S., Eccleston, C. and Williams, A. C. deC. (1999) Systematic review and meta-analysis of randomised controlled trials of cognitive behaviour therapy for chronic pain in adults, excluding headache *Pain* 80, 1–13.

Actual studies and supporting papers

In the present context, a full list of all available studies would be excessive, but the interested reader can contact the authors if they would like further information. The selection presented here includes some of the studies published by the first author as they represent the most direct evidence to support the use of the methods described in this book.

Andrews G. (1996) Talk that works: The rise of cognitive behaviour therapy *British Medical Journal* 313, 1501–1502.

Bendix, A.F., Bendix, T., Ostenfeld, S., Bush, E., and Anderson, A. (1995) Active treatment programs for patients with chronic low back pain: a prospective, randomized, observer-blinded study *European Spine Journal* 4, 148–152.

Fishman, B. and Loscalzo, M. (1987) Cognitive-behavioral interventions in management of cancer pain: principles and applications *Medical Clinics of North America* 74, 271–287.

Frost, H., Klaber Moffett, J.A., Moser, J.S. and Fairbank, J.C.T. (1995) Randomised controlled trial for evaluation of fitness programme for patients with chronic low back pain *British Medical Journal*, 310, 151–154.

Johansson, C., Dahl, J., Jannert, M., Melin, L. and Andersson, G. (1998) Effects of a cognitive-behavioral pain-management program *Behaviour Research and Therapy* 36, 915–930.

Keefe, F.J., Caldwell, D.S., Baucom, D., Salley, A., Robinson, E., Timmons, K., Beaupre, P., Weisberg, J., and Helms, M. (1996). Spouse-assisted coping skills training in the management of osteoarthritic knee pain *Arthritis Care and Research* 9, 279–291.

Keefe, F.J., Caldwell, D.S., Williams, D.A., Gil, K.M., Mitchell, D., Robertson, C., Martinez, S., Nunley, J., Beckham, J.C., Crisson, J.E. and Helms, M. (1990) Pain coping skills training in the management of osteoarthric knee pain: a comparative study *Behavior Therapy* 21, 49–63. (1990) Pain coping skills training in the management of osteoarthritic knee pain II: follow-up results *Behavior Therapy* 21, 453–457.

Kraaimaat, F.W., Brons, M.R., Greenen, R. and Bijlsma, J.W.J. (1995) The effect of cognitive behavior therapy in patients with rheumatoid arthritis *Behaviour Research and Therapy* 33, 487–495.

Loscalo, M. and Jacobsen, P.B. (1990) Practical behavioral approaches to the effective management of pain and distress *Journal of Psychosocial Oncology* 8, 139–169.

Lindstrom, I., Ohlund, C., Eek, C., Wallin, L., Peterson, L. And Nachemson, A. (1992) Mobility, strength and fitness after a graded activity programme for patients with subacute low back pain: A randomized prospective clinical study with a behavioural therapy approach *Spine* 17, 641–652.

Mayou, R.A., Bryant, D.M, Sanders, D., Bass, C., Klimes, I. and Forfar, C. (1997) A controlled trial of cognitive behavioural therapy for non-cardiac chest pain *Psychological Medicine* 27, 1021–1031.

Molloy, A.R., Blyth, F.M. and Nicholas, M.K. (1999) Disability and work-related injury: time for a change? *Medical Journal of Australia* 170, 150–151.

Nicholas, M.K., Wilson, P.H. and Goyen, J. (1991) Operant-behavioural and cognitive behavioural treatment for chronic low back pain *Behaviour Research and Therapy* 29, 238–255. (1992) Comparison of cognitive-behavioural group treatment and an alternative non-psychological treatment for chronic low back pain *Pain* 48, 339–347.

Vlaayen, J.W.S., Haazen, I.W.C.J., Schuerman, J.A., Kole-Snijders, A.M.J. and van Eck, H. (1995) Behavioural rehabilitation of chronic low back pain: comparison of an operant treatment, an operant cognitive treatment and an operant-respondent treatment *British Journal of Clinical Psychology* 43, 95–118.

Williams, A.C.deC., Nicholas, M.K., Richardson, P.H., Pither, C.E., Justins, D.M., Chamberlain, J.H., Harding, V.R., Ralphs, J.A., Jones, S.C., Dieudonne, I., Featherstone, J.D., Hodgson, D.R., Ridout, K.L and Shannon, E.M. (1993) Evaluation of a cognitive behavioural programme for rehabilitating patients with chronic pain *British Journal of General Practice* 43, 513–518.

Williams, A.C.deC., Richardson, P.H., Nicholas, M.K., Pither, C.E., Harding, V.R., Ridout, K.L., Ralphs, J.A., Richardson, I.H., Justins, D.M. and Chamberlain, J.H. (1997) Inpatient vs outpatient pain management: results of a randomised controlled trial *Pain* 66, 13–22.

Williams, A.C.deC., Nicholas, M.K., Richardson, P.H., Pither, C.E., Fernandes, J. (1999) Generalizing from a controlled trial: the effects of patient preference versus randomization on the outcome of inpatient versus outpatient chronic pain management *Pain* 83, 57–65.

Appendix 2

ACTIVITIES

Creative activities
- Doing artwork
- Pottery, ceramics, etc
- Knitting, needlework, sewing, etc
- Taking a course in a creative skill (eg art, photography, cooking, pottery, etc)
- Cooking something special or new
- Redecorating a part of a room or house
- Restoring furniture, antiques, etc
- Woodwork or carpentry
- Repairing things
- Working with machines, engines, electrical equipment, etc
- Photography
- Writing
- Thinking up or arranging songs or music
- Singing
- Playing a musical instrument (alone or with others)
- Learning to play a musical instrument
- Acting or taking acting lessons
- Participating in an organisation related to your creative interests
- Reading books, articles or magazines related to creative interests

Entertainment activities
- Watching television
- Listening to the radio
- Listening to music
- Going to a play
- Going to the movies
- Going to a concert, the opera or ballet
- Going to an art gallery, a museum or an exhibition
- Going to a rock concert
- Going to a sports event
- Going to the races (car, boat, horses, etc)
- Reading the newspaper or a magazine

Educational activities
- Reading books, plays, poems, etc
- Reading about a subject which interests you
- Going to lecture courses or other classes which interest you
- Learning a foreign language
- Learning to do something new (eg acquiring a new skill)
- Going to the library

Physical activities
- Playing bowls or other lawn sports
- Swimming
- Going for a walk
- Snorkelling
- Boating
- Hunting, shooting, archery, etc
- Fishing
- Bushwalking or exploring
- Camping
- Sitting in the sun

- Being at the beach
- Driving a car or riding a motor-cycle
- Going for a trip on a bus, ferry or train (just for fun)
- Participating in a club related to your own sporting interests
- Playing sport in competition
- Playing snooker, pool, etc

Social activities

- Writing to or recontacting an old friend
- Telephoning an old friend
- Visiting a neighbour or friend
- Inviting a friend or neighbour to your place
- Having a friend or neighbour to lunch or dinner, or to morning or afternoon tea
- Arranging or going on an outing with a friend or neighbour
- Arranging a meeting or outing with several mutual friends
- Having friends or relatives over for lunch or dinner
- Throwing a party
- Meeting someone new of the same sex
- Meeting someone new of the opposite sex
- Joining a club (social, recre-ational, academic, etc)
- Going to a wine bar, coffee shop, hotel, etc
- Going to a restaurant with friends
- Going to a party, picnic, barbe-cue, etc
- Being with people you like
- Talking about your interests: sport, movies, politics, philo-sophy, etc
- Going out on a date
- Going to a ball, dance, etc

- Complimenting, praising or thanking someone
- Doing something positive for someone (eg offering assistance, giving a gift, etc)
- Having your preferred sexual activities

Miscellaneous activities

- Active involvement in politics, community or social action groups, etc
- Being involved in religious or church activities, etc
- Speaking a foreign language
- Playing chess, draughts, etc
- Playing cards, bridge, board games, etc
- Collecting things (eg stamps, coins, wine, etc)
- Gathering natural objects (eg flowers, rocks, driftwood, etc)
- Gardening, caring for house-plants, etc
- Visiting interesting places out-doors (eg the zoo, reserves, parks, riverside, harbour, etc)
- Caring for or being with animals or pets
- Being in the country, the moun-tains, or at the seaside
- Planning or taking a holiday or trip
- Giving or receiving massages or backrubs
- Going to a sauna or doing health-related activities
- Having your hair done or cut
- Taking a hot shower or bath
- Getting dressed up
- Having a hot drink in bed at night
- Having a take-away meal
- Having a meal in a restaurant
- Buying something special for yourself (or someone else)